THE
BRAILLE
ENCYCLOPEDIA

Advance Praise for
The Braille Encyclopedia

"*The Braille Encyclopedia* shimmers—poetry in paragraph form. Compelling, often humorous entries show declining vision along with acute awareness. Readers meet Louis Braille and Adjustment to Blindness Training and a braille Torah that isn't kosher because it must be touched. By the end, we understand what 'touching my reading' means. 'When it's so much work to write a single word,' Cohn explains, 'it had better be worth saying.' Cohn's words are worth saying."

—Ranae Lenor Hanson, author of *Watershed: Attending to Body and Earth in Distress*

"Naomi Cohn's *The Braille Encyclopedia* is a story of a life told in moments, in asides, in meditations, in lyric observations that can be as nuanced as they are sweeping. There is an impressive unity to this collection and a momentum that casts a spell as the pages turn."

—Ilya Kaminsky, author of *Deaf Republic*

"Naomi Cohn's engrossing debut memoir *The Braille Encyclopedia* is a wonderful wide-ranging rendering of a life in love with words and the world words make. Cohn brilliantly twines personal and familial history with the history of Louis Braille and his life on the way to creating a tactile language for people living with blindness. At turns poignant and humorous as it chronicles Cohn's progressive loss of sight, I finished this abecedarian collection of essays and prose poems gratefully feeling I'd gotten an 'all-around education.'"

—Sean Hill, author of *Dangerous Goods*

THE

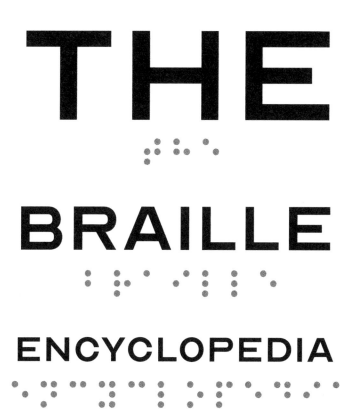

BRAILLE

ENCYCLOPEDIA

Brief Essays on Altered Sight

BY NAOMI COHN

Rose Metal Press

2024

Rose Metal Press, Inc.
P.O. Box 1956, Brookline, MA 02446
rosemetalpress@gmail.com
www.rosemetalpress.com

Library of Congress Cataloging-in-Publication Data

Names: Cohn, Naomi, 1963- author.
Title: The braille encyclopedia : brief essays on altered sight / by Naomi
  Cohn.
Description: Brookline, MA : Rose Metal Press, [2024] | Includes
  bibliographical references.
Identifiers: LCCN 2024028713 (print) | LCCN 2024028714 (ebook) |
ISBN 9781941628331 (paperback) | ISBN 9781941628348 (ebook)
Subjects: LCSH: Cohn, Naomi, 1963- | People with visual
  disabilities--United States--Biography. | Vision disorders--Social
  aspects. | Blindness--Social aspects. | Braille.
Classification: LCC HV1792.C563 A3 2024 (print) | LCC HV1792.C563
(ebook) | DDC 362.4/1092 [B]--dc23/eng/20240624
LC record available at https://lccn.loc.gov/2024028713
LC ebook record available at https://lccn.loc.gov/2024028714

Cover and interior design by Heather Butterfield

This book is manufactured in the United States of America and printed
on acid-free paper.

In memory of my parents, Rella and Barney,
with gratitude for all the ways they
keep showing up in my life.

Table of Contents

Academia................1

Awl........................3

Between..................4

Blind......................5

Blinds....................7

Blood.....................8

Blue......................10

Body......................11

Braille...................12

Button...................14

Cell.......................15

Cindy....................17

Cobbler.................18

Code.....................20

Common Pillbug....21

Contraction..........23

Diagnosis..............25

Dictation...............27

Dot.......................29

Drawing................30

Dream...................31

Error.....................32

Evil Eye.................33

Eye.......................34

Eye Chart..............35

Fifteen..................36

Finger...................37

Fissure..................39

Flower...................40

Focus....................41

Gadget..................43

Glance...................44

Grid......................46

Hinge....................48

Homophone..........49

Ice........................50

Impossibility.........51

Jardin des
    Plantes.............53

Jealousy................54

Kindness...............55

Kitchen Counter....56

Knife.....................57

Knowledge............58

Legal.....................59

Lens......................60

Letters..................61

Library..................62

Line......................63

Literacy.................64

Location................65

Marriage...............66

Memory 68
Mirror Neuron 69
Motivation 70
Mutual 72
Needle 73
Noise 74
Nothing 75
Obituary 76
Occupation 78
Ointment 79
Out of Print 80
Oyg 82
Poetry 84
Pressure 85
Proof 86
Punctuation 87
Quandary 88
Quipu 89
Raphigraphy 90
Reading 91
Repeat 92
Slivovitz 93
Smell 95
Synesthesia 96
Tapping 97
Thread 99
Torah 100
Touch 101
Umami 102

Unforgettable 103
Unseen 104
Village 105
Visual Acuity 106
Voice 107
Window Seat 108
Woman in Blue Reading
    a Letter 110
Work 112
Xerophthalmia 113
X-height 114
Yahrzeit 115
Yearning 117
Yellow 118
Zoom 120
Zorro 121
Zutz 122

Author's Note 125
Notes 131
Sources 141
Acknowledgments 147
About the Author 151
*A Note About the
    Type* 152

Academia

The world into which I was born. Not my world now. But raised among the faux-Gothic towers and gargoyles of the University of Chicago by a linguist mother and a cultural anthropologist/historian father, I grew up in a nest feathered with words, texts, and books.

I am made of words, the organized chaos of text, ant colonies of characters streaming over paper, each letter coalescing into ever greater meaning with its sisters. I am made of words, of the syllable-song of speech, the badminton of argument batted back and forth over the remains of dinner across that round Formica table of childhood. My very cells built of words, the milk and Cheerios and brown sugar, the peanut butter and jelly, the corned beef, bagels, and sardines, lox and cream cheese, Morbier and Manchego, Gruyère and Gorgonzola, all bought with the dollars my father made from words (something like $12,000 the year I was born). Words—read, said, written, and argued.

The milk of words—ethnography and kinship, semester and sabbatical, primary source, archive and field, research, thesis, dissertation, Festschrift and symposium, caste, colonialism, taboo—all churned into the butter on our bread. We got splinters from the aging maple floors of our Hyde Park apartment while my father paid the mortgage with words.

My mother's milk was also words—linguistics and semantics, etymology and syntax, grammar and glottal stop. Reading the dictionary for dessert. And inside my mother's cells, flecks of Yiddish, and potato peelings—scraps of my grandmother's words—stories of a Lithuanian shtetl, of fleeing pogroms, Bolshevik Revolution, World War I—my mother's mother's words, words of a grandmother I never met: *We ate potatoes. We slept on sacks of potatoes. We wore potato sacks for clothes when the potatoes were gone.* In such a teeming ocean of words how could I know there was anything else to swim in?

Awl

A tool for piercing holes, particularly in leather. A simple metal shaft. A knob of wood for a handle, polished by its fit in the sinewy cradle of a leatherworker's palm. Likely the tool with which Louis Braille (1809–1852) blinded himself as a child in France. An accident in his father's saddle-making shop, in the early years of the nineteenth century. Braille later invented a system of raised dots as a means of reading and writing for the blind. We don't know much. Whether he was in the shop with his father or snuck in alone. Whether it was damp and rainy or whether the sun shone and brought to life the floating dust that always hung in the air. Perhaps it was just a little poke in the eye. A small tool, a small slip of the hand, a small injury. How a little fumble ends in blindness. Decades before general anesthetic or antiseptics, the resulting infection spread to the uninjured eye. Perhaps the doctor they rushed him to believed in the value of "laudable pus" in a wound. I don't want to picture it. Did young Braille already know the names of the parts of a saddle—cantle, pommel, stirrup, tree? Did he know the smell and feel of each grade of leather? Of all the tools—punch and pincers, gouge and groover, chisel and awl—the child chose awl. Perhaps the last thing he saw, a shine of metal galloping toward his eye. Is it an accident that my tool for making hand-punched braille is so much like an awl?

Between

From Old English, *in the space which separates*. As in the space between two lines of braille. The inability to move easily from one line to another separates me from a competent braille reader. To me, the interstices feel vanishingly small. Line often separates poetry from prose, line being a tool that poets often use, that prose writers, mostly, do not. I live lost in the few millimeters between lines of braille, lost between poetry and prose, lost in the zone between total sight and total blindness. A whole country that seems invisible to other people, an unimaginable Narnia, as elusive as the space between two lines of braille.

Blind

Blind alley	a dead end
Blind pig	an illegal saloon
Blind drunk	what you get there
Blind staggers	a disease of horses
Blind story	floor of a building without windows
Blind spot	where the car lurks in the next lane

Total blindness is complete lack of visual perception. No sense of light—unless implied by heat. No visual sense of movement. No color, depth, or shape. Less than 15 percent of legally blind people are totally blind.

For many years, my obscure retinal condition failed to render me any kind of blind. I described my eroding vision as *illegal blindness*. Legal blindness is all about determining whether a person is considered sufficiently damaged to be eligible for certain benefits. Measured by how big a slice of the world one can see: visual field. Or how sharply one is able to see that world: acuity.

The legal definition of blindness misses most of the lived experience of altered sight. There are many ways of not seeing. Demonstrations of retinal degeneration often show a calm blank circle at the center of a photo or video. My experience is something like that and nothing like that. Each blind eye, each blind mind, is different.

Blind	screen that hides the hunter
Blind	flying without instruments
Blind	trust
Blind	ambition, rage, fools

Each of my eyes bears its own unique shape of retinal scar. The scars are not silent. My brain supplies a constant message of visual sizzle. A noisy, demanding sparkler. Northern lights. Pain-in-the-ass. Dead center in my field of vision. Dead center, blotting out the letters of a text or street sign or pill bottle. Blocking faces and expressions. If I close my eyes, I still see images of scintillating scars. I do not often see them in dreams. I love sleep.

Blinds

As in shades, a form of window treatment my mother favored over curtains. Not cheap vinyl, but something with a burlap texture, coated, stiffened into respectability. The shade my mother preferred was beige, paper-grocery-sack beige. Beige everything—blinds, woodwork, walls—in that long slingshot of a South Side apartment. To see the light outdoors, you gave a just-so tug and release to the shade, which rolled up, sliding back into itself. A beige snake coiling. Except, if you tugged too hard, the shade snapped and rattled as it thrashed against itself. My mother always seemed to hear, all the way at the other end of the apartment, half a city block away. And what of the broken shades, where the snake refused to budge? The blind creature wouldn't eat its own tail, no matter how you tugged.

The view wasn't much—fire escape, garage roof, iron theft-prevention bars. To the west, the grimier side of Hyde Park and then Woodlawn. Beyond that, the stockyards, unseen. But on an August day, the thick greasy stink of slaughterhouse carried miles to our open windows. How could such a heavy stench float?

One night, decades later, age thirty, soon after I got the diagnosis of progressive retinal decay, I dreamt of an old beige window blind rolling up to a view of nothing.

Blood

That life-giving liquid destroyed my sight. New capillaries nudged their way into the tissue of my retinas. *Neovascularization,* doctors called it; resulting from the progression of my extreme nearsightedness. Tiny blood vessels growing, piercing the layers of the retina. Painless blood needles fraying the fabric they stitch through. Growing in the dark, then bleeding into the eye. A green cloud obscuring my vision. I don't know why I saw this blood glowing green. When I prick my finger, blood seeps out a canonical bright red. But green was the report my brain registered at each misguided leaking capillary. Each new stitch by a blood needle released a new green cloud. Each time, over time, my body re-absorbed the hemorrhage, cell by cell.

Each time, my vision recovered somewhat as the green cloud receded. Until the next time. Each time, a few more cells died, each eye coming to host a dead zone, an unseeing spot. A little blot. Each blot grew. Cell by cell, rod by cone, the capillaries—blood needles—broke my sight. Not all of it. Just a few millimeters of tissue that provided the physical basis of my central vision.

At the time of my diagnosis, no one could give me answers as to why an eye becomes so elongated that it tears itself apart. Even today I have only guesses. A lifetime of increasing nearsightedness, a genetic inheritance from my parents. Or being raised in a bookish, academic community, an inheritance expressed in close focus, head bent over book or paper, rarely breaking away to the long view. Whatever the forces at work, for a quarter-century, starting at age four, my prescription grew stronger. My glasses grew thicker. Unseen, my eyes grew longer. Ultimately this shapeshifting stressed the eye, in my case stretching and damaging the retina and my central vision.

So much of my identity had grown from that central vision. At least until age thirty—with glasses—sighted. One who noticed fine detail: a painter, sculptor, print-maker, quilter, an addicted reader of print, a bird-watcher, a finder of missing commas and extra typographical spaces, a finder of small things dropped on a dark floor. Heady, bookish, precision-oriented. Then one day, a "disease process," long present, long unfolding, but long unseen, announces itself, pokes its way into my retinas.

Blue

Color, as in pigment or light. A color I still see, unless it shades toward midnight, which my eye reads the same as black or dark brown or green. I walk out of the house on a bright blue-sky day, and harsh sunlight teases apart color threads—black, blue, brown, green—that my eyes, inside, read as one color. Possibly my favorite blue is the jacket of Vermeer's *Woman in Blue Reading a Letter*. The woman is a pillar of blue in a composition of rectangles—map, chairs, table, the folds of the letter in her hands—all given their place by light streaming in from an unseen window. The world of the painting weights toward earth tones. Then at the center there is the woman's blue jacket: layers of transparent pigment that read like layers of light. Blue. The blue of a Heavenly Blue morning glory. Created by glazes of ultramarine, from Italian oltramarino, *beyond the sea*. A pigment made from ground-up lapis lazuli. An extravagant, expensive pigment. A pigment made from the earth that reads like the sky.

Body

The rest of the body works to compensate for what the eye can no longer do. A constellation of degenerated disks twinkles in my neck and back from years of vulturing my nose ever closer to printed page or screen. Headaches pulse through some years or decades, recede in others. Double vision. Spasmed muscles. All for the glimpse of letters, characters, or notes on a stave of music. A kind of tired that feels like most of my trillions of mitochondria have decided they've cooked their last energy-meal, turned off the stove, hung up their aprons, kicked off their pinching shoes, and gone to lie down somewhere. For a very long time.

Braille

"Braille," if capitalized, refers to Louis Braille, the child of a nineteenth-century saddle-maker in Coupvray, France. Braille, who accidentally blinded himself with an awl. Braille, who invented a tactile system of reading and writing for the blind.

Lowercase "braille" refers to the system he created. Translating the experience of reading and writing braille into printed word stumps me. I have struggled to write this piece for months. I keep getting bogged down in providing information: Braille's biography, when Braille invented braille, the intricate mechanics of reading, writing, and producing braille.

What I want to write is a love poem. What I felt about books was passion, desire, love. My love of books was a young love, a first love. Visual. Yes, touch mattered, stroking the typographic scar of each letter on a page. But all those beauties in the bookstore! Once I had chosen, I loved to gaze on the beloved.

Large print, small print, the print on cereal boxes, the fading print of cheap paperbacks, the glossy ink of coffee table books. Yesterday's newspaper, microfiche, card catalogs, scribbled notes, hand-painted signs peeling in the sun, maps. A map, its fusion of image and text and symbol.

But now I am older and blinder, and I love braille. I love braille in the way of the old. Loving touch, lights on, lights off, eyes open, eyes closed. It does not matter. I've fallen hard. It's taken years to begin to know the bumps and oddities. The lighter my touch over braille's contours, the more I understand.

When I began learning braille as part of Adjustment to Blindness Training in 2010, people often said that more than half of our brain is allocated to processing visual input. Others said that learning braille uses brain space and neural connections in the visual cortex. New connections reach across, fingers of axon touching fingers of dendrite. Old love wipes out young.

Visual pathways once said *eyes crinkling without a smile* meant *repressed laugh*.

Thick line along seam of t-shirt meant *inside out*.

Thread loose on button meant *find a needle*.

Now I have re-wired. One combination of bumps says *J*. Another indicates a number sign. Feeling the two next to each other now means the clump of dots that read as *J* will now read as *zero*. After much practice, pathways take in clumps of bumps and know: *CH* and *E* and *F*, and recognize *chef*.

It's too much to explain. You know how love is. The intimate knowing defies description. How do you talk about where joy happens?

Braille is the ceiling of the Sistine Chapel, those almost touching fingers of God and Adam. When my finger touches braille bumps, something moves in me.

Button

Something that falls off clothing. As a sighted person, I sewed entire quilts by hand, piece to piece, patch to patch. Stitch by tiny stitch. Even blind, it is ridiculous to pay someone to sew on a button. Ridiculous, too, to give away clothes for the lack of a single button.

But seeing well was useful for sewing well. Small acts turned into intricate art forms. The threading of a needle became a performance in itself. I still sew on buttons. After the fact, I notice that the thread I thought was black might be blue, suddenly shining in October light.

Even if I get the color right, sometimes little loops of thread—dark thread against dark button—have eluded me. Those few millimeters stand and catch that light. Or tying off a knot, I leave two long bristles. Or another knot I didn't tug snug wags like a dog's stumpy tail.

Cell

The blood of language moves through the word "cell," from monk to prison to biological. Braille is composed in cells, units that contain up to six embossed or raised dots, in different configurations, denoting letters, letter combinations, symbols, and, sometimes, whole words. I don't know why a braille cell is called a cell. I don't know how many blood cells Louis Braille lost when the awl he was playing with as a child slipped.

Red blood cells live a hundred days before they wear out from their silent hustle—pounded through the heart's chambered cathedral, rushing out to the farthest reaches of the body with the good news of oxygen.

A red blood cell is measured in microns. A solitary prison cell is measured in feet. As in six by nine. Or less. I don't know what the unit of measure is for how living in solitary changes a person. We know that living in a confined space, without access to the long view or landscape, changes the eye. For lack of practice, the eye loses its ability to make out what lies in the distance. I don't have a unit of measure for what this does to the heart.

A braille cell is measured in spaces in a grid—two across by three down—that can be filled with a raised dot. Imagine this cell as an egg carton that can hold half a dozen eggs. And the eggs, depending on the quantity and where you place them in the carton, can mean different things.

The oldest cell I find in the dictionary is monastic, a place for contemplation. From the concealed place where wine was stored. As in cellar. I find braille contemplative. My hand advances left to right, the touch receptors in my finger triggered by the uneven contact of paper and skin. Messages run along nerves, finger-to-brain, brain-to-finger. Cognition sizzles. My mind notices this feels different from the pathway of sound in ear to auditory processing. Listening pulls me into the world in an infinity of directions. Touching my reading educates me on my place in the world, feet in shoes, weight of foot on ground, weight of bones and flesh in chair.

Cindy

My braille teacher when I was completing Adjustment to Blindness Training, in my late forties. Cindy, my guide from the lowercase letter *a*, a single dot in the upper left corner of a two-by-three grid of dots, through *z* and beyond, into reading and writing so-called Grade 2 or contracted braille. Grade 2 braille makes use of close to 200 shortcuts, which—if you can remember them—save space and reading and writing time. Cindy, master of all the arts of teaching a subject few want to learn: long chats about hobbies, frequent breaks, ready access to the candy jar. Cindy, who can teach two students at once, reading two texts, one with her left hand, one with her right. Cindy, who can read a bit of braille upside down, like Django Reinhardt playing guitar upside down or behind his back. Cindy, who has a particular gift for listening to the stories. New vision loss rehab students usually have their story—how they lost their sight, what they did for a living before, the spouse who left after. Cindy, who has a very gentle way of breaking bad news.

Cobbler

A baked fruit dessert with a thick, pebbled crust. Perhaps it gets its name from its bumpy surface, resembling a street paved with cobblestones. Cobbler, more commonly: a person who makes or mends shoes. My shoes often demand the attentions of a cobbler. The man who repairs my shoes holds up my boots, points to the worn heels and the toes of the sole. He tells me the wear pattern shows I walk too fast. *Slow down,* he says. *Relax. What's your hurry?*

I walk fast because I was the youngest of four children; I had to keep up. I walked to school. I walked to Hebrew school, to pottery class, to 31 Flavors in Harper Court. I walked to the grocery store and the pizza place and to my friend Sarah's in the rain. I grew up in places it wasn't safe to dawdle.

I walk fast because I don't see well enough to drive. I walk fast for the same reason people drive fast: they have places to get to, too many things to do in too few minutes. I walk fast because I live in a climate where winter is long and subzero temperatures remain common despite climate change. Still cold enough, as my father liked to say, *to freeze the balls off a brass monkey.*

I walk faster with my white cane because it tells me things my eyes do not. In winter it growls over concrete (*go fast*), hisses over ice (*go slow*), and gurgles through a puddle (*go around*).

I've worn down the tip of my cane more than the heels of my boots. I notice this quickness with a cane bothers some sighted people. Do they think blind people are supposed to be slow?

Code

In developing his system, Louis Braille was inspired by a military code of raised dots for passing notes. *Night writing,* they called it. This sounds romantic, occult, like dream work. But it might be no more than something that can be shared in the dark, without revealing location or other information. Something the enemy cannot hear. Writing in the dark, in a code almost no one understands, has freed up my writing in ways I did not expect. Braille conceals. Chances are the bumps that mean symbols and words to me mean nothing to you. Or mean something else—mystery, curiosity? Something opens up in the place of concealment. In the silence of the braille cell, I write what I would never put into print.

Common Pillbug

Armadillidium vulgare, otherwise known as the common pillbug, wood louse, roly poly, or doodle bug. Not actually an insect, but a land crustacean. *Vulgare,* as in *common; Armadillidium*, as in *armadillo,* which the little creature calls to mind. They both have armored plates and roll up to protect their softer undersides. A rolled-up pillbug is much larger than a braille dot. I remember, in my four-year-old palm, how the round bead of rolled-up creature unfurled and tickled my skin as it brushed its fringe of legs across my hand. One tactile experience in a sea of visual orientation.

I remember, as a child, holding my mother's hand in an elevator at the Marshall Field's department store in downtown Chicago. I remember other passengers, women in full-length mink coats, something beyond my family's more threadbare economy. I reached out to stroke the soft pelts on those strangers. My mother whispered, *We shouldn't touch other people's thing*s. I still see the minks' dark glisten, the women towering, encased inside their glossy pillars of fur. But I've lost any sense memory of the touch.

But, even today, if I dig just a bit, poke around at the damp margin of a flowerpot, I feel memory pillbugs. The brushstroke of their maze of legs.

In 1967, my family lived in Palo Alto while my father was on sabbatical. Age four, I already had my first pair of glasses, pink faux mother-of-pearl cat-eyes. Merely myopic, preparing for a sighted life. Cross-legged on the ground in the backyard, I sat in the sun, poking between pavers to find pillbugs. I liked their armor's dryness, the feel of each ridged plate, as the curled-up bug lay in my cupped palm, rolling along the track of my life-line. The touch came after waiting: the bug unlocking itself, then the soft legs brushing my hand as it trekked back to dirt.

The visual memories of that California house have faded, dun and dust. But across half a century, the pillbug emerges fresh. Like a braille dot, something closed and round under my finger that—with patience—opens up.

Contraction

Not the muscular pain of labor. A series of symbols in the braille code, shorthand for words and letter combinations. When I began learning braille, there were close to 200 contractions. Each had rules about whether they could stand alone or at the beginning, middle, or end of a word. The day Cindy first slid a model of a braille cell across the table, I felt six dowel-rod pegs fit into a board with six holes. The thing felt like something made in sixth-grade woodshop, the pegs smoothed off, as much by the touch of braille-learning hands as by rough sanding.

Cindy pulled out all the pegs but one, in the upper left corner. This is lowercase *a*. Adding a peg in the hole below it makes the *a* into a *b*. Moving that peg to the upper right makes the *b* a *c*. Then we moved to real braille on paper. Each dot millet-sized and delicate. We spent whole lessons just getting the feel of it, how not to crush the symbols under a searching finger. I learned the alphabet. I learned punctuation, numbers.

I learned whole-word contractions, letters that stand for words. *B* stands in for *but*, *C* for *can*...

> *Do. Every.*
> *From. Go.*
> *Have. Just.*
> *Knowledge.*
> *Like. Many.*
> *Not.*

Cindy jollied me along. *Only 150 more contractions to learn. Oh yes, there is that little matter of learning to get from one line to the next. It is a lot. Would you like another Tootsie Roll?*

Learn new things. Forget old ones. This learning and forgetting is measured not in hours, not weeks, but in months, years. Pack another elephant in the suitcase; you can remember one more thing. Sometimes it is not forgetting, just overload: your fingers move, your brain comes to a halt. By the time I've memorized all the contractions, the Braille Authority of North America has changed the rules and outlawed nine. Through all this slow terrain, no one was as sweet as Cindy, listening to our stories and sliding another impossibility across the table. She knows many of her students do not want to learn braille. Do not want to need a way to read without sight. Do not love its lumpy, clunky difficulties. Do not care to join the 10 percent of blind people who are braille literate. But Cindy still makes the offer. Again and again.

Diagnosis

There are so many different ways of becoming blind.

When I sat at the lunch table at Vision Loss Resources, on any given day fellow vocational rehab students might have reported, in turn, something like this:

Diabetes.
Car crash.
I was a premie and got too much oxygen in the incubator.
Ocular melanoma.
Retinitis pigmentosa.
Accident.
It's genetic.
A tractor fell on my head.
Untreated pneumonia.
Diabetes.
Mystery—I had a headache for nine months. It was my optic nerve.
Motorcycle accident.
Diabetes.
Autoimmune disease....really they don't know.
Got punched in my good eye.

Conditions with labels, but no explanations. Why one eye sees and another does not.

It's different for each of us. Losing sight drip by drip. Rod by cone, axon by dendrite.

Or losing it all at once.

Most blind folks start life with sight and lose it somewhere along the way. But some are born blind; they might argue with my sense of loss. Others go blind as infants or toddlers. They may lose other things—hearing, the parent who died in the car crash, their ability to remember much.

Every body wants—and loses—something different.

Dictation

Not as cool an alternative to sighted typing as you might think. The technology has improved so much since I first tried it back in 2011, in the form of expensive Dragon NaturallySpeaking software. My vocational rehab counselor at the time, who needed his own alternatives to typing, swore both by and at it. Nowadays, speech recognition is built into almost every device. But it still doesn't always get things right. When I dictate:

The Complete Book of Menopause

into a note on my phone, it types:

The Complete Book of Men.

And then pauses.

This moment, multiplied, speaks to my relationship with technology, gadgets, devices. Simultaneous irritation and gratitude. Amazement and amusement.

When I started to lose my ability to read print in the 1990s, it was long before Kindle, Audible, or podcasts. The era of personal computers was just dawning. JAWS and other text-to-speech programs that convert text into an accessible, auditory experience were in their infancy.

So back then, even as I explored the alternatives—cassette tape recordings of volunteers reading books and magazines, commercial audio recordings, audio lecture series—I clung to books. To cloth bindings and shiny dust jackets. To colorful covers of paperbacks. To the brown mildew spots on a treasure found in the free bin at Powell's. To gilt edges. To marbled endpapers. To scalloped indents on the glorious, fat dictionary. To English, French, German, Italian, running west to east. To Hebrew letters clomping east to west. To sifting my right hand along the pages of the future as my eyes shuttled across and back the text, and so down the page, in the physical quiet moment of reading—hands on paper, body curled on bed or carpet or chair or beach blanket—and, at the same moment, fully in the world of the book.

Dot

Spot, as in a dab of paint. Speck. Fleck. As in that first fleck of blindness in my field of view, all those years ago. By the time I moved to Minnesota in 1996, I had a blind spot in each retina and my visual acuity could no longer be corrected to 20/20. By the time I met my now-husband, Ray, tandem biking in 1998, those spots had expanded a bit. He can't see them, but he's never seen me without them.

Ray refers to braille as dots, as in, *Are you off to read some dots now?* A braille dot under my index finger walks up my neurons to some arrangement of synapses, moist like damp leaves, and tickles its way back into meaning.

Drawing

When I was young, I spent hours sketching self-portraits. A mirror is cheaper than hiring a life model. The fallacy of visual art—that delineating the exact surface of a thing can capture its depth. I aged out of drawing, aged out of staring at the reflected folds and puckers of my brown irises holding open black pupils. Decades blink past and today in the cellar, hunting for something else, I come across an old sketchbook and a former self, young and sighted, stares out. Constituent atoms of self shed on Clark Street and Cornelia and Wayne. The Chicago El trains I rode long since decommissioned. That old self, and both banks of the Chicago River with its muddy footprints of raccoons and the tail marks of gravid snapping turtles, long since washed out to the Gulf of Mexico. Standing in the cellar, holding this sketchbook, dusty and soft, I feel I can see the whole image of this old self. It is a mere perception of perceiving. The center of my retinas retired years ago. How can I possibly make out the detail of charcoal eyelash, of dark iris ringing darker pupil? A memory of seeing stirred by touching the page?

Dream

Going blind in midlife is an education in dream deferral. It's not the physical loss, those few millimeters of my central retina destroyed by the growth of a few errant blood vessels. It's only partly the occupations and aspirations that suddenly seem impractical—working as an editor or electron microscopist or set designer, kayaking solo around the Great Lakes, driving a bus, browsing the coupons in the paper, driving to the convenience store. It's also giving up bench presses and aikido, because the specialist suggests they might present a risk to my already threatened retinas. It's the loss or alteration of a thousand pleasures: Flirting across a crowded room with a quirk of half-smile and wink. Movies with subtitles. Reading the whole menu. Window shopping. Each more or less frivolous. But over time, their cumulative diminution takes a slice out of you.

In vocational rehab, each of us has a public dream, an occupational goal, the one we talk about with our State Services for the Blind employment counselor. In 2010, my stated dream was to become a licensed family therapist. It seemed like a listening career perhaps more compatible with my waning eyesight. Very soon, my real dream became gaining enough fluency in braille to read and write it. I ached to reclaim a way of writing by hand. I dreamt of keeping a journal on paper, of jotting notes I could stick in my pocket. I yearned for a way of reading that wasn't a noise—a recorded human or the synthesized syllables of a computer converting text to speech.

Error

In the late 1980s, I worked as a copy editor, proofreader, and fact checker for the *Encyclopædia Britannica*. My one brief corporate job. I earned my bread and butter by finding the widows and orphans, the third *s* nestled like a cancer cell in *confession*. *The Chicago Manual of Style* was our prayer book, a typo a sin. To this day I cannot place a comma outside a closing quotation mark without a pinprick wince.

I was the sort of person who turned off the grammar function in word-processing programs, because I was more highly trained than the software. This is a fact. What is a fact? These are troubling times for facts, but let me offer a fact-checker's answer. When I worked at *Britannica*, a fact was defined as something that could be verified by three reputable published sources. In the late 1980s, in *Britannica's* annual supplement, it was a "fact" that writer Bruce Chatwin died of a rare fungal disease contracted on his travels. I made this a "fact" that found its way into print because I found this information in three *Britannica*-accepted sources. This "fact" was, in fact, a lie. He died of AIDS.

It has been a shift of many years to become a typo-accepting person. To become, in fact, an engine of error.

Evil Eye

Malevolent glare, curse, or what an amulet is believed to ward off. An amulet like the Turkish nazar, a blue-and-white glass disk depicting a stylized, staring eye. My diplomat uncle, my father's brother, gave me one in 1992, after my aunt died. Part of a trove of things they collected—from the 1950s into the 1970s—during their stints in Paris, Islamabad, Kabul, and Istanbul.

Did that eye ward off trouble? It didn't save my aunt from dying of a perforated bowel. It didn't keep me from significant vision loss. It didn't avert my father's twelve years of unraveling through dementia, losing every ability and pleasure that mattered to him. And let's not even start on the state of the world.

But of course, we can't know what additional evils that amulet averted.

Eye

Remember dissecting a sheep's eye in high school biology? Not memorizing the parts—sclera, choroid, cornea, aqueous humor, iris, lens, vitreous humor, optic nerve, retina, macula, fovea, rod, cone—but the rubbery exterior hardened from floating in formaldehyde, the gush of gelatinous matter once a fumbling scalpel finally pierced the tough white sclera and its fine tracery of blood vessels? Remember how gorgeous it was, that butterfly-wing iridescence of retina?

Eye Chart

An eye chart so often begins with *E*.

The most common eye chart is the Snellen, created by Dutch eye doctor Herman Snellen (1834–1908) in the 1860s. Starting with a single letter on the top line, it has eleven lines, with increasing numbers of letters in increasingly small type.

In my thirties, when my retinas began to fail, my memory remained obnoxiously competent. I didn't even work to memorize the eye chart. Nothing to look at in those quiet exam rooms but black characters on a white background. The letters memorized themselves.

This standard eye test, in my experience, also lacks real-life usefulness. As my vision degenerated, kindly eye doctors and their technicians never rushed me in my efforts to "pass" an eye test. Which scares me a little now, thinking about the days when I could still legally drive in Chicago based on my ability to read some line on a perfectly still eye chart in a well-lit room.

Fifteen

At age fifteen, I was wearing glasses with lenses with a correction of negative fifteen diopters. A diopter is a unit measuring the power, or focusing strength, of a lens. Like other myopic, or nearsighted, people, the unadjusted focal point of my vision falls short of my retinas. Nearsighted folks who can afford glasses or contacts get a prescription for concave lenses that subtract focusing power. The larger the number, the stronger the correction. If I understand this correctly, my range of perfect focus at age fifteen, without a prescription, instead of being clear and focused at twenty feet, was focused around three inches. Today, with the progression of my nearsightedness, my prescription is as strong as negative twenty-two, but with my blind spots it's impossible to accurately measure.

At age fifteen, I had no expectation of becoming blind. Retinas still healthy, with fifteen diopters of power subtracted from my eyes, I passed, legally and socially, as sighted. Unless I took my glasses off, like when I was swimming. In a pool or pond or Great Lake, I was suddenly a creature of loose visual impressions, of vibration, pressure, chlorine or algae smell, of sound and light bouncing off water, drip, splash, echo.

Louis Braille left his village home at age ten. At age fifteen, he had been at the school for the blind in Paris for five years and had already devised the key features of his system of reading and writing for the blind.

Finger

Finger, as in the Sistine Chapel God reaching his divine digit to Adam. Finger, as in, *I fingered the culprit*. As in, *Glenn Gould fingered a difficult passage in the Bach prelude*. As in, *I finger the fine silk*. When I do this last one, my fingers—roughed up by running over the openings in the metal braille slate—snag the fibers, pulling fine threads I can feel but not see.

I read braille with the curve of my fingertip, midway between the nail and the central whorl of my fingerprint, as I was trained. That spot remembers the callous from playing a stringed instrument. That spot remembers smudging out an errant line of charcoal in drawing class decades ago. These days, the whorled patterns blur from decades of nicks, cuts, pokes, and burns.

What my fingers have learned about braille unsettled my reading of Anthony Doerr's 2014 *All the Light We Cannot See*. I enjoyed the novel, set in World War II, when I read it soon after learning the rudiments of braille. My reading speed at the time clocked in around forty words a minute, so I was no expert. But I knew adept braille readers mostly used both hands, sometimes just a few fingers, sometimes eight digits galloping over the lines. Having come to braille late in life, my fingers will never be that skilled. But I knew nobody read braille with ten fingers, using their thumbs. So when one of Doerr's characters, a young blind girl, repeatedly reads this way, it sounded jarringly wrong.

It felt wrong as I tried it. When I attempted Doerr's arrangement, my fingers protested. The tendons in the back of my hands and forearms twanged like over-tightened fiddle strings. Suddenly, my fingers were en pointe, the apexes of my fingertips not broad enough to read a whole braille cell, my nails scraping and erasing the dots.

I released my thumbs, let my left hand float away. Relief. My fingers slid back to their accustomed curve. The dots, not too damaged to be read, began to release meaning back into my skin.

I don't mean to point the finger at Doerr. There are limits to how far we can imagine into each other's experience. Sometimes we fail. We are not gods. We reach toward each other with words—outstretched like fingers.

Fissure

A crack, split, crevasse, narrow opening, a long thin line of breakage. As in those thready capillaries fissuring my retinas, moving me past mere eyestrain and headaches, past my fantastical floaters—that bestiary of ocular flotsam to rival anything van Leeuwenhoek ever saw under his microscope lens—and into blindness. Doctors gave my retinal fissures one of those pointless names: *lacquer cracks*, as if the retina were layers of paint, the varnish beginning to crack with time, spoiling the clarity of image underneath.

Flower

Blossom, expand, bloom, develop. The way braille abbreviations or contractions flow out of each other like clusters of grapes. A single lowercase braille *w*, standing alone, expands into *will*. Add one dot in the right spot in front of *w*, and you get a contraction that blossoms into *work*. Add another dot and *work* grows into *word*. With a *w* and three dots in front, the contraction for *world*. A particular arrangement of seven dots, confined in a mere two braille cells, makes this contraction bloom into the whole world.

Focus

What draws attention, interest, or energy. Something a well-constructed telescope, camera, or eye has or does. From the Latin for fireplace or hearth. By implication, where the eye is at home. Mine's at home looking at demons, at least the ones in Martin Schongauer's fifteenth-century engraving, *The Temptation of St. Anthony.* The saint, a bearded, robed old man, floats in mid-air, claiming the image's center. He's kind-eyed and patient even as the demons rain blows. Other than a rough bit of cliff off to one side, we see no sign of the ground below. Anthony exiled himself to the desert to wrestle with his demons. He felt tormented by laziness, thoughts of women, and evanescent piles of gold.

I know my attention should be on Saint Anthony, but I don't care about him. Schongauer has made the demons so damn intriguing—with their composite persons, bodies of bat and squid, bird and cat and lizard. And that one poor sod with hedgehog torso and fish-face sprouting a long trunk or tube. Poised to whack Anthony with a cudgel, he looks so depressed, I wonder if he has the heart. And the enthusiastic cat-faced one—with squid suckers ornamenting spiny wings, tail, and that ornate anus tilted toward the viewer—seems like she just wants her Friskies.

Is her cat face an evil grin or the rictus of effort? The face we make trying to turn the lid of a pickle jar, when only the bite of sour will get the day's bitter out of our mouth? Or is it the glazed smile pasted on my face when trapped in Walgreens among the bunion and corn pads, listening to the plaint of a woman who has no one better to talk at than me? Maybe the demon feels sad for someone who's mistaken her as kind. Or maybe the demon has her own microbiome of tugging, clawing micro-demons.

Gadget

Device, invention, or piece of equipment. I make it sound as if braille is always an artisanal affair, fingers on paper or punching by hand, like some monk in his cell. But I learned to write braille on a Perkins Brailler, a monstrous typewriter with only nine keys and a probably unintentional steampunk aesthetic. I don't own one. When I borrowed and lugged one home to learn on in 2012, it shook the floorboards as I typed. The magazines I read are produced by institutional braille printers, called embossers, that thunder out pages printed on both sides at once. Braille displays, used alone or connected to a computer, tablet, or phone, allow people to read digital braille files and get a braille read-out of what's on a screen. Reading braille electronically can help an avid reader avoid an avalanche of paper. Even a single braille magazine comes in several eleven-by-eleven-inch volumes, each more than an inch thick. I felt lucky to get training to use a forty-cell braille display in 2014. A decade later, on a good day, when I can remember all the commands I learned and get the Bluetooth connection to play nice with my current device, it's magic. Little pins dance up and down on the refreshable display, forming braille characters under my fingers.

Glance

A swift sort of looking. In "When I Met My Muse" William Stafford says:

> *...every*
> *glance at the world around you will be*
> *a sort of salvation...*

Starting in 2015, I led a long-term writing group at Ebenezer, a Minneapolis senior high rise. My students there ranged from sixty-something Ed to ninety-something Fran. Over time, I started teaching in a variety of community settings, mostly with older adults and other people living with disabilities. I often brought this Stafford poem to my groups.

I love this bit, where Stafford's muse says: *I am your own / way of looking at things,* capturing some of my joy as a teacher, helping people find what inspires them. I often tell students about the background of the word, as in a glancing blow, a lance sliding off armor, cognate with the French for *ice,* which we might recognize in the word *glacier. Glance* carries around in it a violence, a slippy defensiveness, a melting coolness.

Glancing no longer works for me. My eyes still dart but don't take in what they used to. Instead, I assemble assumptions. I expect moving cars in streets. Bipeds usually have heads and faces. Faces usually have noses and lips. Yet why is glancing still my habit? Perhaps because, for so long, it helped me pass for sighted.

Braille cannot be taken in with a glance. With my eyes, I see only paper. Unless I put finger to paper and make contact, I will know nothing more.

Grid

As in the two-by-three grid of a braille cell. As in the Amsler grid, a small plastic card handed to me by the first retinologist I visit in the early 1990s. A white card crisscrossed by a grid of black lines. At the center of the grid, a black dot, a legless spider centered in a rectilinear web. You could slip this card, unnoticed, next to the joker in a deck of playing cards.

I had been sent to the retinologist, let's call him Dr. Schmuck, by my longtime ophthalmologist, let's call him Dr. Mensch, when I still lived in Chicago. Dr. Mensch examined my eyes after I'd complained of a transparent lavender question mark that seemed to hang in the middle of my left eye's visual field. For months.

So quiet in that dark room after the long wait in the hubbub of a hallway turned into a waiting area to accommodate some hospital renovation. Silent, Dr. Mensch conducted a slit lamp exam of my dilated eyes, what I experienced as a familiar thin vertical bar of light passing left to right, right to left in front of my eye. Familiar until repeated again and again, perhaps with an unaccustomed wobble reflecting some movement in Mensch's hand. I heard the soft landing of the slit lamp in its velvet case. He put his head in his hands. Then groaned.

He told me there was some deformation of my central retina, that it was a matter for a specialist. He did not need to say this was not good news. I never saw Dr. Mensch again.

The Amsler grid was created in the 1940s by a Swiss ophthalmologist, named, you guessed it, Amsler. A tidy grid of lines and right
angles and clear borders in strictly neutral Switzerland. Perhaps
the last of World War II unfolding around him. The right angles of
Hamburg, Dresden, Kassel, and Dessau all deformed into rubble.
A pall of crematorium smoke still distorting the skies of Europe.

The retinologist directs me to look at the card every morning.
Close one eye and focus on the black dot. In a healthy eye, the
grid of lines will be crisp and straight. In my eye, the lines bent
and blurred, reflecting changes in the layers of the retina.

Each day, I checked each eye, scanning for any new deviation
from the right-angled norms. Each day, for years.

The purpose, I understood, was early detection of any new
retinal changes. Early detection, we patients are told, leads to
early, more effective treatment. The only problem with this
logic is, that in the 1990s, there was no effective treatment for
my condition.

Nowadays these retinal changes are treated with injections of
Lucentis, Avastin, or Eylea, drugs that slow the growth of blood
vessels damaging the retina. Amsler grids are still handed out
to eye patients, though now they tend to use white lines on a
black ground. There's no evidence this is more effective. White
on black or black on white, using an Amsler grid is about 50 percent effective in detecting retinal damage. Pretty cost effective
if evaluated by the price of that little card. But I felt the price of
vigilance: those years of daily blinking at that grid, hunting for
any new sign of distortion, deformation, oncoming disaster.

Hinge

A mechanical joint. The hardware on which a door or gate hangs and swings open. As in the hinge on a braille slate, a tool for embossing braille by hand. If you are perverse enough to want to learn more than the rudiments—as a forty-seven-year-old, born-sighted, visually-oriented adult—eventually the hinge of a braille slate wings open.

I never meant to learn braille. It was just part of the package of vocational rehab, or Adjustment to Blindness Training: Technology, Orientation, and Mobility, Woodshop, Keyboarding, Cooking, and Tasks of Daily Living. I'd never even thought about the possibility that people wrote braille by hand, until I started rehab. I never meant to start rehab either. I just wanted State Services for the Blind to help me earn a quick little master's in therapy so I could shift to what I thought would be a more physically sustainable way of earning a living as the usefulness of my eyesight dwindled. Annie, my vocational counselor at the time, wisely suggested Adjustment to Blindness Training to bolster my chances of getting through grad school as a legally blind student. *Sure, okay, whatever,* I said. When I learned that braille class was part of the curriculum, I couldn't imagine it would be more than a passing curiosity. But I said, *Sure, okay.* And some hinge within me began to unfold.

Homophone

Words that mean different things, but that sound the same. Words which, unless spelled out letter-by-letter, a computer screen reader for the blind does not differentiate as it converts text into synthesized speech.

The ear cannot distinguish *sea* from *see, knead* from *kneed* from *need*. As in

He likes it when I need him.

He likes it when I knead his shoulders.

He does not like to be kneed in the groin.

Reading in braille allows me to distinguish these meanings; to distinguish between *all* in the sense of *every* and *awl* in the sense of *a small, pointed hand tool for denting or piercing holes, especially in leather.*

Ice

A single slippery syllable, *ice* is a perfect word in lowercase braille, rising up the diagonal slope of *i*, then sliding across the horizontal dots of *c*, before melting down the slope of *e*. I can tell you how *e* is the mirror image of *i*, but the little swoop of feeling under my finger—the tactile pun—is difficult to convey, the way familiar landmarks tell you that you're close to home.

Impossibility

In Lewis Carroll's *Through the Looking-Glass,* the White Queen brags to Alice that she sometimes believes as many as *six impossible things before breakfast,* a good practice for learning braille. If you stick it out, through the alphabet and punctuation and getting from one line to the next, Cindy cheerfully hands you the slate, a piece of metal, perhaps two inches down by eight across, heavy and cool in the hand. You feel the top side as a complicated surface of bumps and rectangular openings, the bottom a regular pattern of indents, in groups of six, two across by three down. On the left, a hinge. On the right, a half-moon dent just the right size for an index finger. Your finger naturally presses against the dent and the slate opens, reveals itself to be two pieces of metal hinged together.

You can now feel the top plate has four rows of openings. The upper surface of the lower plate feels like rows of wells—like egg cartons for little fish eggs in groups of six. The lower plate also has four sharp bumps at its corners. I run my fingers over the metal until they seem to have the iron-tang smell of red blood cells. But it is more than I—with my born-sighted bias—can figure out or describe.

Cindy, still cheerful, slides what she calls a *stylus* across the table. Less than three inches long, it's a plastic knob on the end of what feels like a fat, dull darning needle. A tiny awl.

I cannot figure it out. Cindy demonstrates, clamping a thick piece of braille paper between the jaws of the slate. The four sharp teeth of the lower jaw bite into the paper and with the hinge closed, hold the paper fast. Through the topside openings, she presses dents into the paper. I hear a quick tapping as her expert hand punches. Then she pulls out the paper, flips it, and glides it across the table to me. She has pressed into the paper the letters of the alphabet in braille. It will take me months to get the feel of how to press the correct spot in each cell. But that is not the real challenge, Cindy explains.

You read braille as a bump, a series of convexities. But you make braille as a dent, concave.

So to write braille using a slate and stylus, you must relearn everything back to front. Right to left. Reversed. This is the point when many adult learners of braille leave the room, never to return.

Jardin des Plantes

A French botanic garden in the Fifth Arrondissement of Paris on the Left Bank of the Seine. Founded in 1635 as the Royal Garden of Medicinal Plants. A place Louis Braille visited while a student at the National Institute for Blind Youth, founded by Valentin Haüy in 1785. Braille was lucky in his parents. They believed in his capacities and finagled a place at the Institute for him in 1819. He was lucky not to be born a few decades earlier, before anyone aspired to educate the blind. Otherwise, he might, like many other blind folk of his place and time, have joined the ranks of street beggars.

Lucky child that he was, he was sent off at age ten from his village to the Paris school, damp and ill-maintained, with worm-eaten stairs.

On happy days, Braille and other blind boys, led by a sighted guide, all held a rope and walked from the school to the Jardin des Plantes. There they could let go of the rope and walk toward the scent of a pine. They could feel the heat of the sun on one arm and the shade of a chestnut on the other, or the infinite varieties of bark and leaves—the muscly smoothness of the plane tree, a paper skin peeling off like a poster on a streetlamp after rain, or the long cascading tresses of a willow. They could smell the wormwood, rosemary, and pine resin, each aroma palpable as a firm handshake.

Or maybe the children chased each other, or just rolled in the grass.

Jealousy

Once I heard jealousy defined as possessiveness, grasping too tightly something or someone we have in our lives. Envy, by contrast, is desiring what someone else has. For years I was jealous of my eyesight, anxiously guarding my remaining capacities.

Decades later, I'm sometimes awash in envy. I desire the sense of completeness that radiates from friends born blind. I envy more sighted people who can read the whole menu without pulling out a magnifier or text recognition app on their phone. Who can order the right size. Who can avoid walking into glass doors, even without a white cane. Who can write in a strong, legible hand or do archival research. Who recognize people they've known for years. Who aren't taken for an idiot. Who don't cringe when their three-year-old grandchild asks them to read a favorite story.

Kindness

A kind friend suggests: *Write about compelling strangers.* That glint of connection illuminated in a moment, one stranger's hand gripping another's to step—mind the gap—from brightly painted boat to the salt-stiffened grass of an abandoned island in the Venetian Lagoon. A shaft of sun passes over a landscape, the beauty real. Then gone.

Compelling, but not in the sense of those invisible strangers who design algorithms that compel me to buy a used yak wool cardigan and a pair of paisley-print rubber cowboy boots on ThredUp. Or those unjust justices who stole women's authority over our own bodies. (Lucky me, I don't have a uterus anymore, so I can't be compelled to bear young.)

Rather the compelling connection of strangers' kindness, how kindness intertwines with kinship. Like when I walk to my studio, a half mile from my house in Saint Paul, there's a guy sitting on the ledge in front of the old elementary school, now repurposed as a professional building. His bottle, in its brown paper bag, sits next to him. As I pass, he says, *Can I ask you a personal question?* Then, *Are you blind?* Then tells me about his old girlfriend, a flight attendant who got glaucoma. *And they fired her.* Then he pulls up his trouser leg to show me his prosthetic leg and says, *Being blind, wow, that must suck. Can I give you ten dollars?*

I don't take the money. But the kindness, by all means, I take the kindness.

Kitchen Counter

There's a concept called ambiguous loss—a death where there's no body to bury. As in a loved one missing in action. Or a loss, not through death, but through change. Therapist Pauline Boss developed and popularized this concept in a book of the same name. A few years after my father's dementia diagnosis, I first noticed a copy of the book on my mother's kitchen counter. By this time I had moved to Minnesota, but whenever I visited my parents in Chicago, there sat that book on the turquoise Formica. My mother, who, in my experience, had much greater need for being taken care of than ability for providing care, never read it, never wanted to. But there it stayed.

Knife

From late Old English, *a short-handled blade.* Some accounts about Louis Braille's accident say he injured himself not with an awl, but with a serpette, a kind of pruning knife.

I still use knives, especially in the kitchen. Three decades into the slide away from sight, I still have all the fingers of my non-dominant hand, the one that holds carrots, onions, potatoes, celery for slicing, dicing, mincing. I prefer a quiet knife to the food processor's loud whir, to its winged blades that require washing and handling, lying in wait in a dish drain for the probing finger. What I learned from Darlene in Cooking and Tasks of Daily Living was:

Don't be a show-off, chopping vegetables is not a sport.

Keep the knife point on the cutting board, lifting only the handle end.

Keep the fingers of your holding hand well curled, the fingernails folded toward your sheltering palm. Keep your thumb tucked behind the other fingers. All digits are precious, but thumbs are especially useful.

Knowledge

In braille, this word is contracted to a letter *K* with a single dot in front. We want knowledge. We want to know: What caused this? Whose fault? What I have come to know is: we don't always get to know. Whether it was a toxic breeze from the steel mills. Or a single base-pair change on a stretch of DNA. Or the lacemakers disease, too many hours with head bent too close to my work.

Did the repeated act of being bookish deprive me of being able to read a book? Or was my blindness an early manifestation of autoimmune confusion in my cells?

Over three decades, my medical files accumulate: doctors' scribbles and hand-drawn diagrams documenting slit-lamp exams, retinal images from fluorescein angiograms, stacks of color photo series, flash on flash storming the helpless dilated eye. The most recent layer of data: digital images from optical coherence tomography, light-wave-generated cross-sections of the layers of my delaminating retinas. Over three decades, I hear the same, *We'll have a cure in five to ten years.* Over these three decades, my visual acuity changes, line by line on the eye chart, from 20/20 right eye; 20/40 left, to 20/200 or less in both eyes.

Legal

A legal line cuts between vision and blindness. A person takes certain eye tests. The results become a passport, making one a citizen of one country or another. Read eight small letters on a chart, and one is allowed to extend, for now, a stay in the country of sight. This makes as much sense as saying one side of a fish is in Mexico and the other in Texas. Or shaving a clear-cut line across the forty-ninth parallel. Ravens, smoke from fires, slanting rain, all pass over borders without a thought.

Lens

The focal part of an eye or camera. Vermeer lived in a time and place obsessed with lenses and how they expanded the possibilities of seeing. Astronomers looking into the magnified heavens; van Leeuwenhoek focusing his microscopes onto fabric, pond scum, sperm, spittle. O brave new world, that hath such seething in it. Vermeer likely used a camera obscura to help him see how light worked in his world, expanding what he was able to report to us across the centuries.

For many years, lenses expanded my seeing. Corrective lenses kept me on the sighted side of the boundary line between sight and blindness. Most of my life I wore my lenses as eyeglasses. For a decade or so, I wore little slips of flexible plastic—contact lenses—on the surfaces of my eyes. Each morning, touching a fingertip to the disk floating in saline in its plastic case, picking the sea creature from its sterilized tide pool, dabbing it onto the contour of my cornea.

Amazing, those few years, when my body knew what it was to see without a boundary between the world of central focus and what lay beyond the frame of glasses. At least until my eyes felt dry and the creatures pinched, or slid out of place, or leapt out of my eye, or until I tired of those mornings, dripping from the shower, on my knees, running my fingers over the bathroom floor, searching for the feel of a wet, flexible lens, less resistant than the cool tiles but firmer than a drop of water.

Letters

The kind we write to each other. In our cellar—full of all kinds of hoardings of nostalgia, denial, resistance to change—there's a cobweb-draped box of letters. Letters from friends, their handwriting evolving from round childish cursive to something more spiky and mature. Probably as accurate a measure of time as carbon dating or tree rings. Aerograms, tissue-thin, pale blue. Airmail stickers. Stamps for astonishingly scant numbers of pennies. Many silhouettes of Queen Elizabeth II. My father's postcards from London and Delhi, the Albert Memorial, Tipu's Tiger, Neanderthal dioramas, Mughal miniatures. On the backside, pithy, silly, misspelled messages in his inky squiggles, which disease unraveled over the years. I can no more read the writing on those letters in the cellar than I can make out the words on the paper gripped in the tense hands of Vermeer's *Woman in Blue Reading a Letter*.

With his code, Louis Braille, age fifteen, had given the blind a way to write letters to each other. But it took him another fifteen years to solve the puzzle of creating a way of writing legible to both the blind and the sighted. For students at the Institute for Blind Youth, this was no small thing. Many students couldn't afford to travel home. Some couldn't visit family for years. If they wrote their own letter, they'd be unable to check what they'd written. If they hired a scribe, they couldn't confirm what the scribe had inked. Imagine dictating a love letter.

Library

When young Louis Braille arrived in Paris in 1819 to attend the nation's only school for the blind, the library there consisted of fourteen books. Heavy. The largest weighed nine pounds. He could only read their huge embossed letters by feeling each character with both hands.

Even at the low point of my ability to find alternatives to print, I had access to more than fourteen books. And in the past decade, access has exploded. Eternal gratitude to the programmers of text-to-speech software and the narrators of audiobooks: after all those years in the reading desert, I gratefully gobble up podcasts, audiobooks, Kindle books read with VoiceOver on my phone, *The New York Times* in accessible text-only format, an album liner note captured in a phone snapshot and converted by TextGrabber into digitized text translatable by a screen reader. Many formats no longer require specialized devices or training. Nowadays, there are vast digital libraries of accessible words, more than I could ever read. But these libraries don't have plush chairs or oak reading tables. No Tiffany ceilings or modernist walls of windows. No carrels deep in the stacks. No tempting special collections, museum-lit beyond alarm-wired glass doors. Today, my most visited physical libraries are the little free ones, dollhouse-sized homes for those books and literary journals that still find their way into my life, piling up unread and unreadable.

Line

A heartbreaking stage of learning braille. Before you tackle line, you learn dots. You learn letters. Your brain re-wires to make a set of tactile impressions mean something: *D, do, god, dog.* You start reading the braille information in elevators. (You also, long before the pandemic, start carrying hand sanitizer.) But inevitably you have to get to the next line. A fluent braille reader reads with both hands. There are different strategies, but an elegant reader moves in a fluid choreography: right hand finishing the current line, left hand sweeping back across the page to catch the start of the next. The fluent braille reader readily finds the light track of emptiness between two lines, a flat road between hills, an unnatural evenness. Two hands dancing, away, together, away, together. Lovely. In theory. Years into learning braille, my hands barely know the steps of this dance, clumsy ducklings waddling along the page.

Literacy

Hunting for a half-remembered aside by French anthropologist Claude Lévi-Strauss on the ways literacy and writing serve as forms of control, I come across this:

> *Literacy is a linguistic innovation characteri[z]ed by the encoding and decoding of language into a system of visual signs whose relevance to daily life in most societies cannot be overstated.*

This defines me as, what, post-literate? I can still encode language into visual signs, but I cannot reliably decode them. Standing stumped at a crossroads, unable to comprehend the street signs; or in a public bathroom, unable to read a tiny printed injunction; or sitting at my desk using some obligatory, in-order-to-serve-you-better online system for banking or insurance or medical appointments, trying to make my way through one of those "I'm-not-a-robot" captchas or figure out a text with the requisite numbers for two-factor authentication; yes, all of these bring home to me the relevance of decoding.

Location

A couple years after moving to Minnesota, I bought my first house, all of 700 square feet. Perched on a hill between two grandmother oaks, I loved it. I lived there for almost a decade. Only when I moved to a new house did I realize how much more blind I had become. That move—the bumps, bruises, and burns of life in a new space—moved me, at last, to try vocational rehab, to seek some strategy other than just clinging to eroding sight. I find it funny now, how much of what I took for granted as sight turned out to be other things—unconscious memory of the number of steps from one room to another, how many degrees a twist of my wrist moved the thermostat dial. By ear, by feel, by habit—vision-oriented as I was, I claimed it all as sight.

Marriage

Bond, union. My parents were married for fifty-three years. In the early 1990s, my family started noticing. We noticed my father could no longer tell a red light from a green one. His eyes were fine. We noticed when he asked the same question twice. *How's the weather up there?* A minute later, *How's the weather? How's the weather?*

Soon enough, neurologists gave his collection of growing oddities a name: dementia. It took more than a decade to unravel him to death. It was only months after my father's diagnosis that retinologists diagnosed the visual oddity of that violet question mark in my field of view. I've never really managed to divorce the two events, the two trajectories of unraveling, his fatal one, mine so much more subtle.

By the late 1990s I lived in Minnesota and every visit to Chicago, I found my father more shrunken, more confused. More and more firsts: stutter, silence, fall. The time he disappeared in the Field Museum men's room, I fretted for twenty minutes among plastic dinosaurs outside the gendered MEN door, and at last asked a stranger to retrieve him, zipped, buttoned.

Closer to the end, we sought what remained. Like the time, over dessert at Russian Tea Time, when my mother went on for twenty uninterrupted minutes about the origins of the name Zanvel. Natter, chat, a steady rain of knowledge. My father sat silent, dull, then suddenly leaned forward—a bald old snapping turtle—grinned, showing yellow teeth, and said, *I'm worried about your mother's memory.*

Memory

An alternative to vision. Mine used to be hungrier. I never had a photographic memory, but it was once athletic and ravenous. When my thirty-year-old eyes could no longer read a phone number, I naturally leaned on memorization. Just learned something and remembered. Passwords, birthdays, anniversaries, restaurant menus, poems. Piece of cake, cake my memory would eat.

Now, in my sixties, the Velcro of memory has lost its grip, glutted with lint. This makes learning braille—all its letters, punctuation, symbols, contractions, and their rules for use—puzzling. The mind's memory fails. What takes over? Muscle memory, body memory, skin memory. My fingertip remembers more braille than my hippocampus.

Mirror Neuron

I learned, when training to become a therapist, about neurons hypothesized to fire the same way in our brains when we perform an action as when we watch another perform it. The empathy neuron. Seeing another individual smile, frown, cry, get hit with a hammer, all light up these particular neurons. We are social creatures with neural infrastructure that sets us up for understanding (or at least making assumptions about) each other. Where does this leave me and other blind folk? If I don't see you laughing or crying, do I not care? I am not sure. When I was doing one of my family therapy internships, I had a co-therapist who would kick me under the table if a client was crying. Do I now feel empathy in my shins?

Motivation

If it's so hard, why bother? Why write, for example? Because I'm like that cliff-dwelling worm I'm sure I read about as a kid in that encyclopedia I loved: *The International Wildlife Encyclopedia: An Illustrated Library of All the Animals, Birds, Fish, Insects and Reptiles of the World.* Twenty glorious volumes, from aardvark to zorro, a stumpy mutt-looking canine. All rich with fact and picture. With geographic distribution maps, taxonomic information, and text in three important-looking columns. First published in 1970. The lead author, Maurice Burton (1898–1992), was once the curator of sponges at the British Museum of Natural History. My parents bought me the set in the 1970s, feeding my obsessions with both the animal world and with books. I cooed over koala and kangaroo. I flipped past the slimy hagfish and gruesome botfly with a shudder.

I kept those encyclopedia volumes for decades, the same way I kept the hundreds of pounds of other books I began buying for myself as soon as I had pocket money. Even today, I still have books I bought the year my family lived in England. From 1975 to 1976, when I turned thirteen, we lived in Sydenham, South London. My father, on sabbatical, spent his days tunneling in the records of the India Office Library where he was researching the British colonial enterprise in South Asia. My mother was deep into a yearslong hunt for the origins of the name Samantha. I spent my allowance on Smarties and caramels sold in white paper bags at the sweet shop, Osmiroid fountain pens from the stationers at the end of the High Street, and on books from Kirkdale Bookshop: from *Watership Down* and *The Hunting of the Snark* to *Northanger Abbey*, from more books on animals to *I Know Why the Caged Bird Sings*.

My mother complained of the cost, but my father shipped a whole trunk full of those English books, both his and mine, back to the States when we returned home to Chicago.

I lugged many of those books, and all those that joined them through high school and college and into my twenties, with me through much of my adult life, even after my sight began to make text unreachable. From apartment to apartment in Chicago, from apartment to house to house in Minnesota. Eventually I did my grieving and let the animal encyclopedias and most of the others go.

But I still carried the memory of that coastal worm within me. How it lived by eating its way into a cliff face. Over the years as it tunneled, it grew, boring a wider hole as it lived deeper into the cliff, eating mud and stone. I carried with me the story of how it could never turn around, the tunnel behind it too narrow for its present larger self. The way a writer just has to keep gnawing, writing forward into the future.

Mutual

Shared, reciprocal. Inside the doors of the nonprofit agency where I completed Adjustment to Blindness Training, I had a bond with fellow students. Not exactly friends, but here, week after week, whatever our differences, we all crossed out of the space of our regular lives and met. We ran our hands over each piece—lumpy or smooth—that our classmates had made in woodshop. We ate each other's chili and chocolate chip cookies from cooking class. We sat around the lunch table and shared things we didn't share with family. Public bathroom stories were a favorite. You try finding the seat, the handle, the paper, the tap, the soap, the towels—without looking. Or without touching everything.

Needle

A tool with an eye. But not one that sees. The leaf of a conifer. Anything with a pricking sharp point. Something that pokes at you, like a little sister. As a verb, the action of such a sister.

My blindness pokes me each time the thread holding a button on a favorite shirt frays. Lucky if the button pulls away in my hand. Lucky if I have a pocket to put it in. Lucky I know how to use a needle threader, a diamond-shaped loop of thin wire with a flimsy, dime-sized handle. Picture it: you hold it between thumb and forefinger to poke the diamond loop through the needle's eye, prod the thread through the loop and tug the loop out of the needle. Voila! Threaded needle.

But first you have to find the needle threader in your sewing drawer and to master the feel of the hair-thin wire catching in the needle's eye. It helps to use a bigger needle.

But perhaps the presence of thread through loop is beyond your fingers' feeling powers. Perhaps you still have "residual" vision (as if eyesight were a shampoo you'd been too lazy to fully wash out). So, for now, you can bring the needle about an inch away from your better eye. You roll that eye around, like an aggravated horse, until you catch a glimpse of thread.

Noise

Sound that arrives uninvited. Traffic humming on the distant highway. My neighbor's dogs barking; a stabbing, repetitive, relentless sound—to bark the joy of their lives. The refrigerator groaning for its coils to be cleaned. My husband asking me a question while I have my headphones on, listening to a paragraph of text translated into speech. Spouse and text morph together into noise, and the interruption means I have to start over at the beginning of the paragraph. Not born an auditory reader, I can't disentangle competing threads of sound. My eyes still make out letters and even words, but not with accuracy. Magnification helps, but not much: think of making a small mess into a big mess. So, when I have a lot of reading to do, I listen to the words. But my ears grow tired. Braille, by contrast, is a gorgeous lake of silence.

Nothing

What I see is not nothing. I see light and shadow, many colors, shapes, glares, silhouettes, movements. I see print, but it crawls the page like a roil of ants. I see the endless static projection of neural activity my brain superimposes over the hole in my vision, an iridescent spackle job. I see the moon and sometimes, out in the country, stars. Sometimes I see the dark rims of my glasses; sometimes, they vanish. One winter day it is so cold in Saint Paul, my boot heels ring as they strike the pavement. The noise shakes loose a white movement, left-to-right swoop, a patch of winter sky cut loose in the shape of wings. This is not nothing. This is what I call *hawk*.

Obituary

Louis Braille died, aged forty-three, on January 6, 1852. No one published a death notice for the inventor, teacher, and musician whose lifetime savings when he died—about 900 francs—added up to less than a laborer's annual wages. No public notice reported cause of death as tuberculosis, contracted at the school for the blind where he spent most of his life, first as student, then as teacher. No one named his musical talent or work as a church organist. No one mentioned his birth in Coupvray on January 4, 1809. Or his childhood accident, nor how his father hammered nails in the shapes of the letters of the alphabet into a wooden board, so his blind son could learn by feel. No one reported Louis Braille's feelings about leaving his family at age ten to live at the school in Paris. No one eulogized his writing system, his other inventions, his relationships with teachers, students, friends.

At the time of his death, Braille's system—now used worldwide—was not common in France. It wasn't even officially used at the school where Braille had spent much of his life. In 1840, the code was even banned by the school's new director, Pierre-Armand Dufau, who had finagled the ouster of his predecessor, François-René Pignier. Dufau may have banned Braille's system just because Pignier had championed it. Or because Dufau believed, as was common at the time, that the blind should learn to use writing accessible to sighted folk.

But blind students kept braille alive, passing notes to each other, smuggling precious pages of code. It's not clear what softened Dufau, but over time, the blind students wore him down. In 1854, two years after Louis Braille's death, his writing system was adopted as the official French means of teaching the blind.

Occupation

Job, employment, or how one spends one's time. Thirty years ago, when Dr. Mensch sunk his head in his hands and groaned before announcing a diagnosis, was he, perhaps, mourning my loss of future occupational options?

I can't know what he thought or felt. I don't even know what I felt. Unreliable memories have frayed, the handwriting of journals from that time unreadable to me now. But my guess is: nothing. Numb. Stopped in my tracks, an animal frozen in the glare of oncoming headlights, dazzled.

As to my occupational options: less than half of Americans with a visual disability are employed. Way less. According to the Cornell Institute on Employment and Disability, in 2021, an estimated 33.9 percent of working age Americans with a visual disability worked full-time, year-round. This same source reports that 25 percent of people with a visual disability live below the poverty line, compared to 9.9 percent of people without a disability.

As for me, by the time I was legally blind and qualified for intensive vocational rehab in 2010, I was entirely self-employed. So no matter how little money I made, I didn't count as unemployed.

Ointment

Something a fly gets stuck in. Unguent, healing salve. Meant to be soothing. A balm. In the medicine cabinet, half-used tubes wait, their emptied ends coiled like scorpion tails. A tube of toothpaste and a tube of ointment feel so similar in the hand. Desenex and Colgate feel so different in the mouth.

Out of Print

A quiet *O.P.* or *O/P* penciled on the flyleaf of a book in a used bookstore or on all those volumes on the British Raj my father collected over the years—most bought for a few shillings each on Portobello Road—on his visits to London.

Much of what I've written is out of print. A little chapbook of poems on insects, *Between Nectar & Eternity,* 2013, a letterpress edition by the late lamented Scott King, founder of Red Dragonfly Press. *Voices of the Watershed: A Guide to Urban Watershed Management Planning,* 1999. *The Unofficial Canoe Guide to the Chicago River,* 1996.

Most of what I've written was never formally published: thousands of pages of grant proposals, narratives, and budgets. Program books for concerts. Brochures, white papers, press releases, and public service announcements. Or published, but ephemeral: like issues of *Disclosure,* a newsletter on community organizing, the house organ of National Training and Information Center (NTIC) in Chicago. Decades of writing, reading, and editing. Decades of words, most of them now unavailable.

My favorite piece I wrote for NTIC covered the 1987 protests by the San Francisco branch of ADAPT (which, at the time, stood for Americans Disabled for Accessible Public Transit). These protests were part of a decade of national activism that ultimately led to requiring bus lifts for wheelchairs as part of the 1990 Americans with Disabilities Act. During the protests, wheelchair users rolled their chairs in front of and behind buses en route. They stopped traffic long enough for another protester to get out of their wheelchair and crawl up the steps of the bus, demonstrating the barriers to using public transit. I loved interviewing the activists, but I had no inkling how much their work to make a more accessible world would mean to me in just a few years.

Oyg

Yiddish for eye. As in:

ein oyg es ganz; die andere vet farbesern

or

one eye is perfect; the other will improve.

Family legend claims this is how a Des Moines horse trader, in the early 1900s, replied to my immigrant grandfather, Jacob, when my ancestor protested he did not want to buy an obviously blind horse to pull his brewery wagon. Jacob and the horse trader, the used car salesman of his day, would have bargained in Yiddish, their shared mother tongue.

I never met this Jacob; I construct him from a photo my mother had in her study when I was a child. Her father and her Uncle Jerome pose proudly in front of Des Moines' American Bottling Company, their joint business creation. A wagon and two pale draft horses always drew my eye. The horses' kind ears swivel, forever, toward the camera. A complexity of yokes and harness delineate their well-fed curves. Both brothers sport company caps and full mustaches. I'll say Jerome is the one by the big-spoked rear wheel, in shirtsleeves and a suit vest, holding a crate of bottles. Jacob, in a three-piece suit with a glint of looping watch chain, rests a calm hand on the near horse's rump. The scene is redolent with hops, horse sweat, and the brothers' satisfaction at making something of themselves. Jacob kept the books, calculating the dollars still needed to think of finding a wife.

Likely, no one bought that blind horse. Sent to the knackers with hooves still glossy, belly still griping from the unaccustomed oats it got to eat while the trader tried to sell it. I imagine that horse, yawing its head to gain some smeared, jittery image. The way I catch myself doing.

Poetry

A magazine available in braille as well as on a mostly accessible website. I am so grateful for this that I pay for a paper subscription even though I often don't understand the poems the editors choose and even though I cannot read the print magazine. I stack them unread to give to my students. Other times I tear open the wrapper, smell the soy ink with its mixed notes of soil and factory. I turn the pages and see shapes of things—little couplets like deer tracks mincing down the page.

Pressure

One aspect of the sense of touch. Others include vibration, contact, distortion, tickle. Stretch. Itch. Ouch. All perceived through an ecosystem of specialized sensory receptors: nociceptors collect what the central nervous system labels as pain. Thermoreceptors inform of heat and cold. Mechanoreceptors specialize in distortion and pressure.

Pressure: its theme and variation allow my fingers to read braille. Pressure, along with heat, transforms shale into slate. Pressure. Too much finger pressure crushes paper braille.

Using a fingernail's pressure and movement, scraping away a braille cell, is one way to erase a mistake. Most of what I create in braille is for my brain only—journal entries, first drafts. So I mostly don't bother to open the slate, flip the paper over from writing side to reading side, and apply the pressure needed to erase an error. But I wish all my mistakes were so easy to undo.

Proof

I tear open a foil packet and a cascade of yeast granules hisses into a cup of warm water, tested against my wrist. Yeast, wise little beasts, only work in comfort. The granules ride the surface resistance for a moment, then fall, one by one, into their deep. Yeast wakes up and multiplies.

Proofing: testing the yeast before committing flour and salt, oil and elbow grease to the making of bread. Or perhaps the yeast tests us, decides in its democracy of single-celled sisters whether this house, this kitchen, this bowl, is worthy of its gift of loft to a loaf.

Mathematical proof. How I loved in eighth-grade geometry writing the letters *QED—Quod erat demonstrandum*—that which was to be demonstrated, or proved, underlining the three letters with two firm pencil lines.

But today, I show things to my eyes all day long and they no longer see the proof of it. They cannot glance around the room and confirm that the stove is off, the windows closed, the milk back in the fridge. If seeing is believing, then is blindness doubt?

Punctuation

I learned all the punctuation marks in braille, then forgot most of them. I remembered the comma (a single dot in position 3 of a six-dot braille cell); the capitalization mark (a single dot in position 6); and the ellipses.... I remembered the period, but questioned, did I really need to punch three dots just to mark a sentence's end? When I was first learning to write braille by hand, it was so much work, I'd often leave off even the few marks I remembered. So today when I find something I brailled a decade ago—even if (miraculously!) I'd written 188 characters without any typos—it reads like this:

reading over this braille journal begin to experience the true value of punctuation the way it helps to make meaning the syntax indicate the pause where to take a breath where to break the line

Quandary

Perplexity. Like the evolving dilemma of how to present my work. I tried memorization. I tried writing in forms, so the repetition of a villanelle, pantoum, or sestina might create a scaffold my memory could climb. Large print. Larger print. Grotesquely large print combined with reading pieces over and over in advance, spending hours practicing a five-minute selection of poems.

When asked to be a commencement speaker when I completed my midlife masters in family therapy in 2014, I spent hours making a usable copy of my speech in braille with my slate and stylus. At the ceremony, I marched up in my shiny rented robe with my white cane and recited something encouraging, pithy, funny. How we're all interdependent. Got a standing ovation. The university president quipped I could go into doing stand-up if the family therapy didn't work out.

But that was a three-minute speech. I practiced it so much, I knew it by heart. I ran my fingers over the braille more as reassurance than as reading. Today, a decade after that graduation, my braille reading still isn't good enough to read pages and pages of text as a way of presenting my work aloud.

I will find a way to read this to you. But there won't be any more of opening a book at random, smoothing each page, the left to the left, the right to the right, and just launching into my words.

Quipu

Spanish spelling for khipu, which is Quechua for knot. A khipu is a collection of multiple strings, knotted in specific ways to record information. It dates back in Andean cultures at least 1,000 years. Since string rots more easily than stone or clay tablets, and since the invading Spaniards deliberately destroyed the records of the Inca and other civilizations, it's hard to prove that it was also a writing system. In recent years, though, scholars have been teasing apart the ways khipus conveyed meaning. Khipus likely encoded not just numeric accounting but narrative. Stories were stored in the arrangement of strands, the direction of their twist, the fiber used, the placement and shape of knots. A kind of tactile writing I itch to get my hands on—to feel in my fingers further proof that eyes are not the only way we humans read.

Raphigraphy

Also known as decapoint, a system of writing invented by Louis Braille in 1839. It could be read tactilely by the blind and visually by the sighted. Braille used a grid, ten dots high, to represent standard print letters. The raised dots were legible to the blind; when combined with carbon paper, a sighted person could make out the letters, which look weirdly like something produced on a dot-matrix printer. The cumbersome system never found widespread adoption. What endures for me is Braille's zeal to empower the blind to write their own letters to sighted people, to create that yearned-for conduit of contact.

Reading

When I was in vocational rehab, I read a handbook for blind college students. To be ready for post-secondary education, it stated, one should—along with being able to do one's own laundry—be able to read 300 words a minute in print, braille, or audio. Even today, I probably read fewer than 100 words a minute in braille. When the inhuman voice of my computer reads to me, I can crank it up to 400 or 500 words a minute before it erodes into a barrage of noise spattering my eardrum. The computer reading is nothing like the relationship I had with a bound book. Braille promises the pace and interplay I miss, the pause as an idea lifts from the ground. The impossible helium of an image fills a bag of brilliant silk that didn't exist until I imagined it. Now, tethers loosened, it rises away, the colorful bag against the bright idea, high above the ground, a new perspective. And when I've let the balloon rise as far as I want, I look down at the plaid of streets giving way to the checkerboard of farm fields. However far I've flown, I can land in the precise spot on the page, return to the very letter that launched the reverie. I land and pick up right where the author left off.

Repeat

To do again and again. Over decades I develop arthritis from the origami I make of my spine, especially my neck, as I relapse, repeatedly, in my addiction to seeing print on paper and screen. Contorting my body in my attempts to see or seem to see. A refusal to let go of words on the page. Or is it an addiction to making a living, having a roof over my head, a fridge with food in it? Likely all of the above.

My body also adapts to braille. Calluses thicken on my fingertips from repeated moving touch. My skin brushing, again and again, over bumps of braille printed on stiff paper, the moving pins of a refreshable braille display, the metal openings of a slate waiting for the tap of a stylus.

Slivovitz

An Eastern European plum brandy. I made my first batch in 2015 to salvage our Minnesota plum tree's first crop. I scrounged a recipe online. Slivovitz, like learning braille, feeds on time as well as effort. The brandy requires a minimum of three months to bubble in the dark, which translates into some explaining to Ray. He tolerates my experiments in pickling, but he needs reassuring after he comes across the gallon jar of eyeball-sized orbs floating in blood-tint liquid in the cellar.

It took three years for that plum tree we planted to bear brief white blossoms. Five years before it bore a crop of plums to ripeness. Its thin branches hung to the ground with fruit the size of quail eggs, their indigo skins dusted white, their insides chartreuse. But the taste on the tongue oozed pale and bitter. The idea for slivovitz grew from desperation, the piles of fruit starting to rot on the counter.

How many years did it take for a horticulturalist to come up with a variety of *Prunus* that would self-pollinate and bear fruit in our peach-less Zone 4? When Ray drove the spade into our backyard soil, we found animal bones. How many years did it take for those bones to decay to that rusty orange, for everything else to fall away? What were the chances that enough of my slivovitz-drinking, Yiddish-speaking ancestors would emigrate to America, some time after a stretch of pogroms, but before the Holocaust? A thread of chance lets me remember tiny glasses filled from a round bottle after dinner, guests sipping slivovitz, snipping piles of grapes with stork-shaped scissors, when it wasn't a crime for parents to hand children a thimble of alcohol, fierce and sweet.

When I strain out the plums, their flesh, once queasy green, has flushed to rich red, the influence of those indigo skins. The brandy that remains glows bright red-purple. Nothing like the commercial clear firewater of my youth, this stuff's become its own thing. The plums and sugar and knuckle of lemon skin and spirit and cinnamon stick, rolled tight as a Torah, all evolve, dissolve into slivovitz.

I started learning braille about the same time we planted that plum tree. Five years to arrive at anything like literacy. Another patient fermentation.

Smell

I lost my sense of smell when I got COVID in 2023. Not entirely. Not permanently, but for a few weeks, it was as if my olfactory sense had gotten extremely nearsighted, could only pick up what was right under my nose. And what I did smell was incomplete. I held a bottle of essential oil, peppermint and tansy, half an inch from my nostrils. Tansy tinted the slow liquid a glorious clear blue. My eyes blinked at the menthol, but all I smelled was sweetness. For those few weeks I stumbled around, suddenly more blind, forced to see how much my nose had been filling in for my eyes.

Synesthesia

How I can't hear as well with my glasses off. How it feels foolish to tease apart the threads of different senses, of memory, imagination. How I can't tell you whether I feel or hear the change of texture under my cane from ice to open ground. How I feel I have seen the orange of an oriole when I hear its jazzy call in the cottonwoods. How the smell of wet acorns makes me feel I see their clever shape, their little shaggy berets atop glossy nuts. How ice smells blue.

Tapping

The sound my stylus makes as I write. The sound a wood-pecker makes on the telephone pole in the alley behind our house. Drumming, ornithologists call it. In my Saint Paul city neighborhood, a small tangle of leafy streets pressed between highways and railyards, the noise is most likely made by a flicker or a downy woodpecker. My tapping sounds most like the lit-tle downy. One December day, a loud bird comes through our neighborhood: black, maybe crow-sized. Calling calling calling. Ray and I are walking the ice-slick streets. We follow the black dot. I ask Ray if it has any white on it. Yes, he sees the flash of its wings as it comes to roost in a bare oak. Calling, still calling. Another bird responds. A pair.

Back home, I listen to a birding app. Yes, that is the call. I peer at tiny photos. Yes, that is the white stripe. I piece together a pileated woodpecker. Usually a bird of deeper woods, it's wan-dered here to call among our city oaks. A pileated woodpecker is big enough for me to get an impression of with my naked eye. Memory tells me it looks like a striking dinosaur, flying through the trees. Its hammering echoes across woods. The birding guides show it dressed like a superhero, a white light-ning bolt streaking its black neck.

My stylus noise evokes strong responses. My tapping does not indicate a hunt for food, nor any direct communication. My tapping's just a by-product of my braille writing, a by-product of eventual communication. I remember sitting in the audience at a conference panel, taking notes in braille. A woman in front of me kept turning around, twisting her body with a face even I could see was wrinkled with displeasure. I neither explained nor responded. Likely she had no idea what I was doing, could not identify the slate or stylus, but nonetheless wanted to shush me.

Other times I use slate and stylus in a writing workshop and people come up to me during breaks to tell me how much they like hearing the sound. Usually I smile, but sometimes not. Like a woodpecker, I am just trying to live my life.

Thread

The companion of needle. The fiber that binds up the slashed wound of buttonhole, that gives the button the safety of holding without hand or finger. The warp and the weft, the showy quilting stitches, ant-sized but more orderly. The practical inner work of basting stitch and blanket hem. The through line of a conversation or a life.

What thread connects this life—braille reading, lost button ignoring—to that needle-wielding person that I was? In Greek mythology, three Fates determine the thread of each life. One spins the fiber, one measures the length of our years, and one snips it to end our days. All destined from the outset.

How can my life be one unbroken thread? What still ties me to the myopic copy editor in her twenties or the girl who sculpted a mouse out of a mini Tootsie Roll, the rodent's brown sticky eyes smaller than millet seeds? What ties me to that child who could find her mother's dropped earring back or a needle lost in the cushion of a chair? Is there a fourth Fate, whose time-roughened fingers snag the component fibers of the thread, leaving us tangled or dangling, connected to our past by a single frayed strand?

Torah

Rabbi Lenny Sarko of Pennsylvania may have created, as recently as 2021, the only Sefer Torah, Book of Law, in braille. Hebrew braille, which was formalized in 1944, runs left to right, unlike print Hebrew which runs right to left. The Braille Torah is not, strictly, kosher since it was not made by a traditional Torah scribe and since, to be read, it needs to be touched. Not by a yad or ritual pointer, but by a human hand.

Touch

Mode of perception that does, and does not, compensate for lost sight. The lighter my touch, the more I feel. Touch is easy, even though I grew up in one of those families that was not very contact-oriented. Even though my British spouse often embodies the stereotypes of his culture around physical demonstrativeness. Yet we are frequently mistaken for a touchy-feely couple. We hold hands a lot. People assume we are just that affectionate, but there is something of chicken-or-egg in it. Touch is part of our closeness *and* a lot of our contact starts in the pragmatic. If I don't have my cane out, I take his arm to cross a street. Sometimes the touch of a hand substitutes for the raised eyebrow or other fleeting expression that more-sighted humans use as commentary or cautionary gesture in social situations. Sometimes we are across a room from each other, silent. I sense he's conveying something, the ingrained bodily habit of a half-smile or wrinkled nose. I ask, *What sort of face are you making?*

Umami

The savory, meaty, earthy deliciousness of dashi broth, vine-ripe Black Krim tomato, roast chicken, shiitake, porcini. Along with sweet, sour, bitter, and salt, one of five scientifically recognized tastes. Identified in 1908 by the Japanese chemist Kikunae Ikeda.

Braille makes up the merest fraction of my reading diet. But just as a little gob of miso, a sprinkle of fish flakes, and a thin strip of kombu seaweed can transform hot water into the sustenance of broth, even a tiny dollop of braille brings flavor to my words.

My acoustic reading, by contrast, is a sugar rush of information.

Unforgettable

Right now, in Saint Paul, my neighbor is walking by in what seems to be unforgettable afternoon light with his dog—all golden, lit by Dutch cloud light. What might have streamed into Vermeer's window if we ever had a chance to stand where he stood.

I hope I will never forget looking at the *Woman in Blue Reading a Letter*. Such a small canvas. So much light and shadow.

While I am remembering standing with Ray in front of the painting, looking and looking, the dog has already passed out of my window frame.

The first day the frost is really gone, the ground gives, soft underfoot. It feels unforgettable, how it brings me some fraction of an inch closer to Precambrian bedrock, closer to magma. That first earth-soft day also releases a smell—life, death, funk, compost. Suddenly we remember every walk every neighborhood hound took around this block all winter long. I don't blame my neighbors for not sticking their hands in the iced-over snow to grab a steaming turd. I do have a certain bitterness toward the woman who drives up in the SUV and lets her dog crap on our lawn. Every day. But can I say I will remember it until the end of my days, or the end of my remembering?

I hope not.

Unseen

Not visible, or, perhaps, not noticed. As in, how I no longer notice what my eyes leave unseen. As in mysterious forces at work in the cosmos—gravity, electro-magnetism, love. As in how Ray, private, self-effacing, would rather have remained unseen in these pages. As in a window in a painting, unseen, but implied by light. As in winter sun, veiled by clouds, unseen anywhere in its brief daily arc above the horizon. When, for a moment, the light breaks through, we snap to attention, like dogs, sniffing the air, sitting up for a treat.

Village

As in Coupvray, where Louis Braille was born and buried. One hundred years after his death in 1852, his writing system had been embraced in France and adopted internationally. (As I write this today in 2023, Wikipedia attests to its use in 133 languages worldwide.) In 1952, on the centenary of his death, the French government honored his achievement by entering him into the Panthéon, a mausoleum for distinguished Gallic citizens. The honor required digging up his bones out of the village churchyard. The residents of the village protested this removal of their native son. A compromise was reached. Paris got his body, cremated into ashes. Coupvray, in an urn atop his former grave, kept his hands.

Visual Acuity

Sharpness of vision. Herman Snellen, creator of today's most commonly used test of visual acuity, also created a chart he called the Tumbling E, intended for people "who cannot read and young children who don't know the alphabet." This chart uses lines of ever-smaller capital *Es* facing in different directions. The patient, using three fingers, shows the orientation of the arms of each *E*.

Over decades, the trend line of my own acuity slopes downward through a scatterplot of better, worse, the same. Some days, eye clinic staff resort to testing me on a Tumbling E, making me a companion to the young and the illiterate. Other days, on a standard Snellen eye chart, I can intuit enough of the impressionist blur—a gray houndstooth weave of what I know, but barely perceive, as letters—to pass for 20/200. I cannot break the habit of trying to pass a test.

Voice

After a few years of keeping a braille journal, I notice a different voice emerges. Sometimes wild, sometimes catty, but more and more, a voice that does not pull punches. Not wrapping everything in endless modifiers. When it's so much work to write a single word, it had better be worth saying.

Despite my ready tongue, I have always been afraid to say my mind. But so few people can read what I write in braille. I can leave a screed, a manifesto, or a satisfying string of insults and obscenities face up in the middle of a room.

Window Seat

My favorite place to read or write. As a kid I loved sneaking into the walk-in closet in my father's study. Part of its magic: it boasted its own small window, an open view to the south. Also, no one else claimed it as their particular space. I'd wander in and reach up to tug the long string hanging from the bare bulb and set my book atop the built-in storage shelves. I'd pull out my mother's sewing kit, a toolbox with trays, full of bobbins, thimbles, pins and needles, embroidered name tags for each of her four children, waiting to be sewn into the collars of clothes. I'd run my finger over the spools of thread. Trusty cotton and elegant silk, my mother ordered them into a perfect rainbow, like a new set of crayons not yet jumbled by use. Tucking the kit away, I'd open the skate drawer, explore the tangle of laces and blades, wonder which of my siblings' scuffed cast-offs I'd grow into by winter. Then I'd hoist myself onto the wide shelf, next to my waiting book—*Pagoo, Misty of Chincoteague,* or one of the Narnia Chronicles. Standing, I could read the titles of paperback mysteries on open shelves overhead—*Murder Must Advertise, The Daughter of Time, The Thin Man, Friday the Rabbi Slept Late, Flying Finish.* Then, like a dog settling into her bed, I'd sit cross-legged and peer out at the tennis courts, the gray limestone of International House, the cars all pointed north on our one-way street. Unseen but felt: the Midway, where every year, come winter, its summer turf was iced into a third-rate rink. My father, his high-school-hockey-star status long abandoned, would take me there to mince and stumble until our cold fingers called out for hot chocolate.

Sitting in my window seat, I'd flick my eyes from that view, back to the open page, and join the world of the book in my hands.

Woman in Blue Reading a Letter

I come to look at Vermeer's painting multiple times in 2015, when it is on loan from the Rijksmuseum at the Minneapolis Institute of Art. The woman in blue gets a room all to herself on the main floor. She has her own guard. The first surprise is how many people walk by without even looking. The second surprise is how quickly the ones who do stop to look move on.

The painting measures eighteen by fifteen inches, under glass in a wide gilt frame. Soon the glass and frame recede, and I see a woman with a blue jacket, a map on the wall behind her. Sunlight traveling in from an unseen window. Tall-backed chairs, a table with a sparse scatter of objects.

With my glasses off, the woman becomes a squat blue obelisk. The folds of the letter disappear.

Those massive black chairs, their empty seats and imposing backs, stand guard around her. With my glasses off, the chairs disappear and a black geometry, a play of rectangles, comes forward.

I look with my glasses on and with glasses off. I go home and look at reproductions in books and online, my eye close to screen and page. I come back and look again.

The woman's light brown hair merges with the soft deltas of the map on the wall behind her. The map shows seas beyond seas; she is painted with a pigment that means *from beyond the sea*. People wonder if she is pregnant, wonder if the letter is from—or about—a merchant husband, overseas, perhaps not returning.

I wonder how my loss of visual detail makes colors and shapes speak more clearly to me. Ray, with his clear eyes, sees tiny dabs of paint that mark shiny metal bosses on the chairs' upholstery. I see the black shapes trapping her. I see a painter's joy at the abstract composition of shape and dark and light. Who cares what is on the letter? Look at how Vermeer makes folds with paint. Look at the intensity of his looking, how he chose what to see.

Work

These days, on a good morning, I sit in my improvised window seat. A couple years ago, I bought three reasonably sturdy storage ottomans and pushed them together in front of a southeast-facing window. Tossed a yoga bolster and a few pillows on them. Gained a slanting view of trees and houses facing a pocket park, bordered by the arrow of street pointing to a distant high rise. In winter, up before dawn, I settle on this seat, nestle into the pillows, drape a throw over my legs against the seeping chill. I stare out at the moving glare of car lights. I pull out my braille journal, punch a few lines with my stylus onto a piece of card stock held tight in the jaws of the slate. On good days, life's a braille sandwich: at night, lights out, glasses off, I read a few pages of a braille magazine, the texture under my fingers lulling me to sleep. I rarely read whole books and when I do, it often takes me months. But these bits of braille reclaim my sensory pleasure in reading and writing. And this pleasure, it turns out, is my real work.

Xerophthalmia

Fancy-pants word for dry eyes. An old friend on my list of eye conditions, I've lived with it almost as long as my retinal degeneration. These days, in my sixties, I seem to make a new friend every time I go to the doctor. Meet your cataracts. Meet your friend glaucoma suspect.

X-height

A property of a font or typeface. In print typography, the height of lowercase letters, benchmarked by the letter x. X-height measures the body, or torso, of the letters on a line, setting aside ascenders and descenders. Descenders include the dangling legs of y or g or q. Ascenders are the arms, reaching up from an h or l. For visual readers, x-height in a font matters. Whether in print or on screen, larger x-height generally means greater readability.

It charms me that the height of a typeface is measured by one of its rarest letters. And many languages, like Italian, don't have an x. So does it have instead a quagga-height? A dodo-height?

For me, in braille, the height of letters does not vary. Three dots deep. Braille has no general equivalent to the splendid, diverse array of print typefaces. Braille gains readability from sameness, each cell the same dimension as the first letters and words Cindy slid under my fingers more than a decade ago. Page after glorious page.

Yahrzeit

A candle lit on the anniversary of a death. Tonight it's my mother's yahrzeit. Dead fifteen years. I can't read the prayer book, so I rattle off a string of remembered syllables, all run together like a screen reader. Ray, wearing a kippah stitched by his tailor grandfather, shushes me because it makes him stumble as he reads the Hebrew text from the book.

I didn't inherit my mother's Zionism, nor her almost lifelong belief in a deity. (She said watching what my father went through in his last dementia decade turned her atheist at the end.) What I did inherit was a head full of words: the glorious spendthrift excess of English. We didn't just have a dog, but a hound, a cur, a canine companion. Even today, things my parents gave me fly from my mouth. Funny how many are unprintable. Mother had rules: you could use any of George Carlin's seven banned words, so long as you could define and spell without error. But never, ever, tell someone to *Shut up.* That was rude. My parents also gave me shards of Yiddish—schmuck and putz, shiksa, treyf, and goy. This mother tongue curves more to insult than to praise.

As a family therapist, I learned to hand children a language of feelings: mad and sad and glad and scared. How useful it would have been, when a child myself, to be able to label that strange nondigestive twist in my gut, that pattering heart, that sudden gout of tears triggered without an ounce of chopped onion in sight.

But tonight, watching a quivering flame mirrored on a black window—how does it cast this flicker of presence?—I'm without words.

Yearning

If my mother's been dead fifteen years, that means my father's been dead twenty. So we can never get back that last pastrami sandwich. The one my brother and I smuggled from Manny's after he picked me up at O'Hare on one of our mutual visits back to Chicago. Maybe 1999, 2000. We'd both moved away years before, but sometimes managed to time our visits to our ailing parents to also see each other.

We can't ever feel again that exact heartburn after standing in the Manny's lunch crowd line, after shouting *Pastrami* at the corned beef guy, making him turn his bulk and knives to carve from the peppery slab, after eating both halves and the pickle and the entirely excessive latke, watching the grease from that extra sandwich we ordered speak with a spreading mark on the white deli bag. We can get pastrami. There will be pepper, salt, and fat; meat cured to the color of an heirloom rose. But we can't sit on a lakefront park bench with our father in the August heat as he eats that sandwich, the one we hid from our mother because she wouldn't have approved of all that cholesterol. We can't get back my father eating without dropping one cracked peppercorn, one single caraway seed, though his brain no longer told him where his feet were or his cousin's name. He still knew how to hold that gargantuan sandwich with as much feeling as a blues harp player just before letting loose the most wailing riff. He still knew my brother, who clambered onto the riprap after a swim in Lake Michigan. He offered his dripping-wet child that leftover pickle, glowing in the afternoon light.

Yellow

Light with a wavelength of around 570 nanometers. Yellow pigments come from so many things you shouldn't eat, like cadmium and uranium, one form of which is called yellowcake. When I was little, one physics building at the University of Chicago had a basement corridor with lovely yellow ceramic tiles. According to the technicians who worked there—one of whom was married to my childhood pottery teacher, Dorothy—they were made with a uranium-based glaze that still emitted radiation.

Genuine Naples Yellow pigment was made of lead. Chrome yellow. Yellows from tin and rutile and benzodiazepines. Other than the honest dirt of a natural yellow ocher, all a pretty poisonous lot.

Even if you could find a brilliant yet edible yellow pigment, nothing could beat the yellow of the eggs Ray made me a few days after my abdominal surgery in 2021. Propped up in my tattered robe, I was grateful my decayed vision spared me details of the six-inch incision, covered with its grin of Steri-Strips. Still wobbly from the useful poison of general anesthetic, I wanted none of my usual Sriracha, kimchi, or salsa verde. I declined even black pepper, just wanted salt and scrambled eggs, a fluffy buttery mass on dark pumpernickel. I'm not even embarrassed to repeat the animal grunts of delight over being alive to eat that yellow cloud, to live with a man who knows how to scramble an egg, to still see enough to see the visible yellowness of wavelength reflected back into my eyes.

Yellow, hallelujah. Yellow butter in the pan. Yellow sun clearing my neighbors' houses on a winter morning. Sometimes I stare straight at it, what do I have to lose?

Zoom

My digital camera boasts a 30X optical zoom. With practice and luck, I use it to pull a dark fleck moving through blue sky into a hawk, crow, eagle, heron. But the greater the power, or magnification, of a lens, the smaller the field of view. That bird on the wing passes out of the camera's eye in an instant. It's similar on a computer. On my new laptop, with its built-in accessibility features, I can, with a few keystrokes and finger gestures on the touchpad, zoom in until a single word, *zoom*, fills my screen. But I can't read much this way, even the slightest gesture jerks the powerfully magnified view off-screen. And reading via magnification means constantly zooming in, zooming out—zooming in to decipher some text, zooming out to find some vanishingly tiny icon of three dots that hides all the useful operations I might need to perform. Or having managed to zoom in and fill out all the text fields on a screen—to buy a plane ticket, make a medical appointment, search for a testing or vaccination site I can walk to (answer, there is not one), renew my legal business name, buy a birthday gift for a friend, fill out an application for services, use a financial calculator—I have to zoom out. I have to hunt for the elegantly microscopic *submit* button. More than a few minutes of this and I have to go hunt for the Dramamine.

And as to that video meeting software that took over the world during the COVID-19 pandemic, human contact beyond my spouse became one endless headache.

Zorro

Spanish for fox. A rather unprepossessing South American canine. The last alphabetical entry in *The International Wildlife Encyclopedia,* that twenty-volume set with all the pictures that my parents bought me as a kid. The one I lugged around for so many years before finally letting it go. The one in which I remembered reading about that ever-tunneling coastal worm.

I never forgot that worm. I couldn't remember the creature's name and, with all my decades of research skill and digging on the internet, I couldn't unearth a likely candidate. Time and again I looked. Nothing.

It kept gnawing. One day in 2021, unbidden, the worm showed up in a piece of my writing. Wanting to flesh out the worm memory with some facts, I shifted my hunt to acquiring a replacement set of the books. I found one advertised for over $2,000, another, on Amazon, for $9. Reader, I bought the one for $9.

A big box arrived, with a creak of our screen door, and a thunk on our porch.

I sat down with the volumes. Got out my phone to magnify the list of entries. I flipped through looking for familiar pictures. Nothing. Front to back, back to front. Aardvark to Zorro. Zorro to Aardvark. I never found the worm.

Zutz

A poke or a punch, like the action of making a dot with my braille stylus. From Yiddish, at least as it was used in my family. When I look it up today, I find it's spelled, and pronounced, *zetz*. I guess that's fitting, since my father was never much of a speller. And I hear the word in his voice, his Brooklyn accent still fresh, *Give it a zutz*, encouraging me to shove a little harder on a sticky door.

Braille will not restore my sight. It will not help me grok a pie chart or find the bright red tips on the feathers of a cedar waxwing. It will not confirm my memories: not how individual droplets make up the roar of a waterfall nor how Ray's eyes glow a warm hazel, flecked with darker brown. But learning braille, using braille, even in tiny doses, thaws out something I had to put on ice over the years. Something I lost contact with as my old print-bound ways of loving language slipped from my grasp.

So when Ray wanders upstairs, finds me sitting in that cobbled-together window seat, asks what I'm up to—my right hand hovering with stylus mid-air, my left hand holding my place on the braille slate, but my attention out the window, caught by some shape winging by—I say, *Just zutzing some dots.*

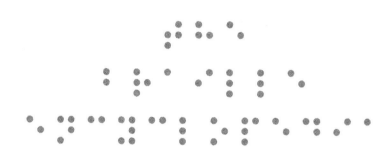

Author's Note

I didn't set out to write an encyclopedia, imaginary or otherwise. Inspiration for the form came from Rebecca Solnit's *The Encyclopedia of Trouble and Spaciousness*. Solnit's book is an expansive manifestation of what nonfiction can be and do, but my initial scheme was specifically inspired by the book's opening essay, "Cyclopedia of an Arctic Expedition," an alphabetical exploration of a trip to Svalbard; I loved how the form, rather than restricting, freed her to move easily from lyric natural history and travel journaling to reflections on human history and climate change.

All I aimed to do was write one essay, maybe a few thousand words, on learning braille as part of adapting to progressive vision loss. In 2015, I'd received a grant to support exploring creative prose after years of focusing on poetry. I quickly gave the piece the working title *The Braille Encyclopedia* as an homage to Solnit's work. The structure of encyclopedia entries gave me a series of smaller vessels to contain my writing, which was useful practically in working with text as a blind person. I also found it creatively useful: The scaffold of the alphabet gave the puzzle part of my brain something to noodle on, while simultaneously providing openings for going deeper into my experiences.

The piece soon expanded into something much bigger than a single essay. Over several years of writing and revision, it morphed into a mix of poetry and prose. When Rose Metal Press accepted the manuscript in 2020, I'd presented them with a collection of what I called linked prose poems. But in revision, it became clear that at least some of the pieces were more solidly prose; Rose Metal not only agreed, but they also embraced the shift and the expansion of the breadth of the book. We've called the pieces "brief essays," but the lines between forms feel flexible, and I'd call some prose poems, lyric fragments, flash memoirs, or vignettes.

The alphabetical encyclopedia form, even though I originally thought of it as a temporary scaffold, has endured through all the revisions. What started as a form of support has become the form itself: the armature has become the sculpture.

So form supports. But form also distorts. No memoir or personal essay can (or should) capture the gestalt of a life. But in weird—and to me, unexpected—ways, the form transformed the content. One aspect of this metamorphosis arose from the demands of filling out the sequence of the alphabet. For example, I wasn't originally planning to revisit the medical journey of my vision loss in this project. I'm more interested in adaptation than diagnosis or, for me, nonexistent treatments. The medical system, doing its best to fix the unfixable, often made me feel like my body and I were a problem. My life got a whole lot better when I focused less on medicine and more on how to adapt, including engaging in vocational rehabilitation, which I experienced as empowering me to live fully in the body I had. But when you're looking for an X for your imaginary encyclopedia, the lexicon of medicine is hard to pass up.

Another example of form distorting is how much Yiddish has crept into this work. I've always identified as Jewish, if nonreligious and non-Zionist. But once again, the ecosystem of the encyclopedia tugged me into exploring my family history and other cultural strands of my life.

But perhaps the most forceful tug of the encyclopedia form is toward a stance of implied expertise. Of facts. Knowledge. Authority. The fiction of being able to be comprehensive about anything. The only authority I fully claim is being expert in my own particular life. I have the greatest fondness for facts and have tried to bolster this imagined encyclopedia with accurate information, but ultimately this is an account—and a fragmentary one at that—of personal experience as I remember it, an inherently fallible source.

A note on altered sight. I'm not—in this book or elsewhere—consistent in how I refer to blindness. I tend to say *I'm blind*, which can be confusing to many people who associate that term with a total lack of visual perception, because, at least as of this writing, I obviously see a lot and am still visually oriented. But to say *I'm blind* is briefer than saying *I'm legally blind (according to definitions used in the United States)*. And I've always found the U.S. definition of blindness weird: as I understand it, in the eyes of the law, I had so-called normal vision until I was thirty, because as long as I wore intensely powerful corrective lenses, my vision was 20/20, meaning that a person can clearly see an object twenty feet away. In a legally blind person, vision is 20/200 or less, or their field of vision is less than twenty degrees. Roughly 1.1 million Americans fit the definition of legal blindness, stemming from cataracts, glaucoma, age-related macular degeneration, diabetes, and other conditions. In addition, the World Health Organization estimates that 800 million people live with vision impairments that impact their daily functioning simply because they lack access to a pair of glasses. So my being defined, and able to function, as *sighted* for so many years had a lot to do with geography, luck, and privilege. But that's usually way more than I want to explain any time somebody asks about my vision. One more observation on altered sight: as much as I like language that centers people rather than conditions, I find referring to myself as a *person living with blindness* cumbersome.

Finally, some other information that might be helpful to readers: The overall eye condition that led to my vision loss, and ultimately to this book, is called pathological myopia. (The terminology is not entirely fixed. It's also been called progressive myopia or myopic degeneration.) Myopia, or nearsightedness, is very common and not, in its simple forms, a particular risk for vision loss. I got my first pair of glasses at age four and I don't think anyone worried that meant I was going to go blind.

But when myopia becomes more extreme, it can place stresses on the eye. As a person grows more nearsighted, the eye itself grows more elongated. The change in how we see reflects an inner anatomical change in the shape of the eye. This shape-shifting, over time, can strain and ultimately damage the eye. The stress can show up in a variety of ways, from retinal detachment and macular holes to damage to the optic nerve and other issues at the front of the eye. In my case, the damage initially manifested in the relatively uncommon form of vascular damage to the central retina. In the ensuing decades, I've moved through the roller-coaster stage of active, acute, and repeated hemorrhages, to the slower motion process of scarring and atrophy.

This progressive and ongoing nature of my vision loss makes it difficult to telescope events into a single representative moment or experience. Running parallel to this, add my many occupational shifts, including working mainly for a variety of nonprofits as an activist, editor, writer; shifting to similar work but self-employed; retraining as a therapist; shifting away from working in traditional therapeutic settings to working as a teaching artist in community settings. And, since the pandemic, increasingly just writing. I won't begin to try to summarize all the print-disability technologies, software, and strategies I've used for reading and writing and making a living over the arc of all those changes. Even over the course of writing and revising this book I've used a variety of strategies, including combining magnification and the VoiceOver screen reader on my Mac and phone, making braille with slate and stylus, and using dictation and the braille screen input function on my phone. Since none of these methods or combinations works perfectly, and since all of them, one way or another, take a toll physically, my other constant companion is a timer, so I limit the increments in which I read or write to limit the wear and tear on my body.

This circles me back to form. All these moving parts, progressive changes, and adaptations make a single, linear narrative challenging if not impossible. But the encyclopedia form generously supports the complexity of my experience. I set out to write one essay about learning and falling in love with braille, about the surprise and pleasure of regaining a means of reading words on a printed page. But I found I needed to write a whole book, not just about braille, but also about its inventor, Louis Braille, about my family, my past, and my efforts to adapt continuously and live fully through all the ongoing changes in my vision. The form invited me to range through all these themes as the right letters and words arose. I make no claims to encyclopedic realism, but hope it makes for an enjoyable read. And I hope, like any good encyclopedia, it satisfies existing curiosities while sparking new ones—whether that's the itch to explore some topic I've only scratched the surface of here, or to learn braille (check out hadley.edu), or to write—past boundaries and categories—into the infinite possibilities of form.

Notes

Awl

Years after writing this piece, I read C. Michael Mellor's *Louis Braille: A Touch of Genius*. Mellor believes the injuring implement may have been a serpette, a sort of pruning knife. But many other sources say awl.

his father's saddle-making shop

Mellor distinguishes between saddle-makers and harness-makers, and Braille's father, living in an agricultural community, was almost certainly a maker of harnesses for farm and other horses. But I've preserved him as a saddle-maker here since that was my first imagining of him based on what I knew when I wrote "Awl."

Blind

Statistics here and elsewhere are generally for the United States.

The legal definition of blindness

According to the Social Security Administration:

> *We consider you to be blind if your vision can't be corrected to better than 20/200 in your better eye. We also consider you blind if your visual field is 20 degrees or less in your better eye for a period that lasted or is expected to last at least 12 months.*

The National Federation of the Blind proposes a more inclusive definition:

We encourage people to consider themselves as blind if their sight is bad enough—even with corrective lenses—that they must use alternative methods to engage in any activity that people with normal vision would do using their eyes.

Blood

extreme nearsightedness

This is called, variously, progressive myopia, degenerative myopia, myopic degeneration, or pathologic or pathological myopia. When I open MyChart in 2024, it says, among other things, "bilateral degenerative progressive high myopia." In addition to the panoply of names for the same condition there does not appear to be agreement in the scientific/medical literature on whether pathologic myopia refers to anatomy, when the axial length of the eye is 26.5 mm or greater, or only to eyes where that elongation begins to manifest in damage to the vision. To further complicate matters, this vision loss can manifest in a variety of ways, including as retinal detachments, macular holes, macular thinning, choroidal neovascularization and subsequent scotomas, or scarring. The impact on the vision is also influenced by the location. Macular or central damage, which is where mine started, is much more disruptive to acuity than peripheral events of similar magnitude. Glaucoma, other optic nerve damage, and cataracts are additional potential sources of vision loss associated with pathologic myopia.

All told the prevalence of vision loss related to pathologic myopia is as high as 2 percent globally.

As to the prevalence of myopic neovascularization in particular as a cause of vision loss, it's not common. According to the American Academy of Ophthalmology, "Myopic Choroidal Neovascularization" occurs in 5 to 11 percent of people with pathologic myopia. Of those only a third develop the condition in both eyes as I did.

It was years before I found another person my age with a similar condition. And the responses of medical staff when I was first diagnosed in the early 1990s bolstered this sense of rarity, or even freakishness, especially in an otherwise apparently healthy thirty-year-old. I remember a medical resident, unconnected with my case or care, sneaking into my exam room to get a peek at the photos of my retinas that were laid out on the desk awaiting the retinologist's appearance. The retinologist's obvious anger at the resident was my clue that the younger man had no business being there. The two men argued in front of me, completely ignoring my presence, and the trainee admitted he just wanted to look at my photos to gain experience with an eye disease he'd never seen.

Braille

Adjustment to Blindness Training

Also called vocational rehab or rehabilitation, I've used the terms interchangeably.

more than half of our brain is allocated to processing visual input.

While it's not stated, the figure presumably applies only to fully sighted people. But it does appear to be evidence-based: According to University of Rochester scientists (cited in a 2012 article by Susan Hagen), more than half the cortex, or surface, of the brain, is involved in visual processing.

Cell

six embossed or raised dots

There are exceptions: an eight-dot cell is used in some technical and computer environments. There have also been efforts to use an eight-dot system to represent Japanese kanji.

denoting letters, letter combinations, symbols

Braille also developed a system for notating music. In the twentieth century, blind mathematician Abraham Nemeth developed a code for representing mathematical equations, adopted by the Braille Authority of North America in 1952 and today called Nemeth Code.

Cobbler

The man who repaired my shoes for many years died unexpectedly in 2022. I will miss him, and not just for his skill with leather. His name was Jim Picard, but he was called Eddie because his shoe repair business, Fast Eddie's, was named after its original owner. RIP Jim, I will try to go easy on my boots.

Eye Chart

Information about the Snellen eye chart comes from the American Academy of Ophthalmology webpage, "Eye Chart Facts and History."

The letters memorized themselves.

Nowadays it's common for the letters to be projected from a computer through a mirror, so the chart doesn't have to be twenty feet away and the doctor or technician can change the letters. But in my experience, they often don't bother.

Gadget

Another recent braille device is my smartphone, which lets me tap braille onto my touchscreen, translating the symbols to English letters and words. When in braille input mode, my iPhone lets me tap braille on the touchscreen using the same fingers I'd use on a Perkins Brailler or braille notetaker—left index for position 1, left middle for position 2, etc.

avalanche of paper.

According to what I've learned informally from more expert braille users, braille usually runs at least three pages to a print page. Technical writing, which may make use of Nemeth Code to represent equations, can run as much as twenty-five braille pages to a single print page.

forty-cell braille display

Like much other braille technology, braille displays are not cheap, usually costing several thousand dollars. By contrast, I bought my braille slate for about ten dollars. As of this writing, you can get one for less than twenty bucks.

In 2020, the National Library Service for the Blind and Print Disabled (NLS) announced the rollout of a free braille e-reader. It doesn't have all the features of a more advanced braille display, but it's a leap forward in terms of affordable, portable braille access.

In terms of the other devices mentioned in this piece, a Perkins Brailler costs about $800. Braille printers or embossers, tend to run to thousands of dollars, with institutional-level embossers running as much as $80,000 or more. Among my braille-using acquaintances, I do not know anyone who has a home printer.

Grid

Dr. Schmuck

Okay, so schmuck is an overstatement. It's not really personal, more an expression of frustration at the limitations of the medical approach to vision loss. The system is not well-designed to connect patients to practical resources.

To give one example: Damage to the macula or central retina impacts depth perception, and losing depth perception impacts all kinds of activities, from close work to navigating stairs, curbs, and other changes in footing. But in thirty years, no medical practitioner ever mentioned this information to me; I first learned it from Kelly, my orientation and mobility instructor, about fifteen years into living with the situation.

Another instance is that, in my experience, eye doctors don't mention or appear to know about vocational rehabilitation resources. I'd been experiencing a level of vision loss that qualified me for vocational rehab for years before any eye specialist mentioned it. And when it did happen, many years after I'd needed it functionally, it came in the form of a clinic receptionist handing me a printed packet after a visit. I was fortunate not to have waited for the medical system to offer that information. I recently learned that in Minnesota eye doctors are required by law to provide this information, so perhaps that stimulated the production of the packet.

drugs that slow the growth of blood vessels

Avastin is a cancer treatment that inhibits the growth of blood vessels in tumors, and is used off-label for eye conditions, the goal being to inhibit the growth of new, noncancerous but still destructive capillaries that damage the retina.

Even when these drugs became available, no doctor suggested I try them, presumably because the damage to my retinas was already too extensive. Even if they'd been available from the first detection of my retinal degeneration, it's unclear how much, if at all, they would have stopped or slowed the destructive process. Whatever the case, I'm glad not to have been poked in the eyes with a needle every month for thirty years.

Knowledge

20/200 or less in both eyes.

I'd guess my acuity is more like 20/400 or less, but how much my neurons are capable of filling in my visual gaps varies enormously. My vision also varies day to day, even moment to moment—depending on light conditions, physiology, and mysteries of the universe.

Literacy

The quote comes from Claude Lévi-Strauss' memoir, *Tristes Tropiques,* pages 391–393, as cited in Mary Kalantzis and Bill Copes in "Lévi-Strauss on the Functions of Writing."

Motivation

An Illustrated Library of All the Animals, Birds, Fish, Insects and Reptiles of the World.

I adore the grandiosity of that title, as if humans could even come close to knowing all the creatures of the world.

Obituary

But blind students kept braille alive

It's not clear how Braille himself responded to this situation. While he was still teaching for at least some of the years of the braille code ban, I did not find any information about his own attitude toward it. Since he was in increasingly ill health due to tuberculosis and needed to stay in Dufau's good graces to retain his position, I suspect he would not have directly challenged it.

Occupation

without a disability.

Many advocates for the blind estimate unemployment rates of 70 to 80 percent. From my own observations, it's clear that more profound blindness, on average, equates with more profound unemployment. But it's maddeningly hard to find accurate, current data that teases apart legal vision impairment and "low vision" from legal blindness.

Out of Print

volumes on the British Raj

After my father's death in 2003, my mother donated most of my father's collection of these mostly nineteenth-century books to special collections at the University of Chicago library. I kept a few random selections: *The Revelations of an Orderly* by Pounchkouree Khan, 1866, as well as *The Tiger of Mysore: A Story of the War with Tippoo Saib* by G. A. Henty, no publication date listed, but first published in 1896. I kept this one to learn more about Tipu Sultan, a staunch opponent of the British who commissioned a mechanical tiger devouring a British soldier that my father had introduced me to as a tween when we lived in London. The tiger is still on display at the Victoria and Albert Museum. As to the book, from peering at a few lines, it's clear it is so appallingly biased that even if I could read all the print, I couldn't bear to read it. And *Tales of the Punjab, Told by the People* by Flora Annie Steel, 1894, which I admit I kept for the engravings and fancy gold tooling on the cover.

Oyg

Oyg is also transliterated as *aoyg*, but spelling, schmelling.

Jacob, in a three-piece suit with a glint of looping watch chain, rests a calm hand on the near horse's rump

After writing this piece, I learned from a brief biographical note my mother wrote about her father before she died that it was likely the other way around: my grandfather Jacob in shirt sleeves and Jerome with his hand on the horse's rump in the photo and also the one who may have negotiated with the horse trader. But there's no one alive left to ask.

Pressure

erase an error.

Another technique is to overwrite a mistake by filling all six dots of a miswritten cell. This can be confused with the contraction for *for,* but context is king in reading braille.

Quipu

Daniel Cossins' article "We Thought the Incas Couldn't Write. These Knots Change Everything" in *New Scientist* provides fascinating detail about khipus.

Stories were stored in arrangements of strands, the direction of their twist, the fiber used, the placement and shape of knots.

Color and color patterns were also visual ways information was encoded into khipus.

Torah

Most of the information for this piece comes from Justin Vellucci's June 1, 2021 *Jewish Chronicle* article, "Local Rabbi Creates Braille Torah for the Visually Impaired."

Umami

Ikeda (1864–1936) was also one of the fathers of modern junk food: According to Wikipedia, he isolated and developed industrial-scale processes for producing the umami-flavor enhancer monosodium glutamate, or MSG. Yum.

Visual Acuity

Information about eye charts from the American Academy of Ophthalmology webpage: "Eye Chart Facts and History." The quote: "who cannot read and young children who don't know the alphabet" is also from this source.

Woman in Blue Reading a Letter

Some people are obsessed with debunking Vermeer, dismissing his art because he may or may not have used technology, the camera obscura. But for me that's not the point. He chose what to include in the frame.

Sources

I've included below a list of works referenced, but for those curious about specific topics, here's a little general information for further reading:

Blindness

Both the National Federation of the Blind (NFB) and the American Foundation for the Blind (AFB) have useful websites.

Louis Braille, His Writing System, and Other Inventions

C. Michael Mellor's *Touch of Genius* is the most detailed source I found. The Musée Louis Braille website was also useful, as were conversations with braille users and teachers I've had the privilege to cross paths with.

The NFB and AFB websites as well as Hadleyhelp.org contain other resources on braille.

Disability

Cornell University's Yang-Tan Institute on Employment and Disability provides statistical information on work-related aspects of disability.

Medical Background

The American Academy of Ophthalmology has a number of online resources, especially EyeWiki. The National Library of Medicine was another useful source.

Perception and Senses

Ed Yong's *An Immense World: How Animal Senses Reveal the Hidden Realms Around Us* is a great read and a trove of information. The BBC podcast *Made of Stronger Stuff* was another engaging source. And anything by Oliver Sacks.

Vermeer

I found Laura J. Snyder's *Eye of the Beholder: Johannes Vermeer, Antoni van Leeuwenhoek, and the Reinvention of Seeing* transformative; I also relied on Jonathan Jason's *Essential Vermeer* website.

Yiddish

I used YIVO Institute for Jewish Research and the Yiddish Book Center websites, as well as Leo Rosten's *The Joys of Yiddish*.

Works Referenced

"Blindness and Vision Impairment." *World Health Organization.* 10 Aug. 2023, www.who.int/news-room/fact-sheets/detail/blindness-and-visual-impairment. Accessed 26 Feb. 2024.

"Blindness Statistics." *National Federation of the Blind.* January 2019, nfb.org/resources/blindness-statistics. Accessed 9 Feb. 2024.

Boss, Pauline. *Ambiguous Loss: Learning to Live with Unresolved Grief.* Harvard University Press, 2000.

Burton, Maurice, and Robert Burton. *The International Wildlife Encyclopedia: An Illustrated Library of All the Animals, Birds, Fish, Insects and Reptiles of the World.* Marshall Cavendish Corporation, 1970.

Cohn, Bernard S. *An Anthropologist among the Historians and Other Essays.* Oxford University Press, 1987.

Cohn, Bernard S. *Colonialism and Its Forms of Knowledge: The British in India.* Princeton University Press, 1996.

Cohn, Bernard S. *India: The Social Anthropology of a Civilization.* Prentice Hall, 1971.

Cohn, Rella. *Yiddish Given Names: A Lexicon.* Scarecrow Press, 2008.

Cossins, Daniel. "We Thought the Incas Couldn't Write. These Knots Change Everything." *New Scientist,* 12 Jan. 2022, newscientist.com/article/mg23931972-600-we-thought-the-incas-couldnt-write-these-knots-change-everything. Accessed 18 Feb. 2024.

"Disability Statistics." *Yang-Tan Institute on Employment and Disability.* Cornell University, disabilitystatistics.org. Accessed 19 Feb. 2024.

Doerr, Anthony. *All The Light We Cannot See.* Scribner, 2014.

Foer, Joshua. *Moonwalking with Einstein: The Art and Science of Remembering Everything.* Penguin Books, 2012.

Frith, Margaret. *Who Was Louis Braille?* Penguin Workshop, 2014.

Hagen, Susan. "The Mind's Eye." *The Rochester Review*, March-April 2012, University of Rochester, www.rochester.edu/pr/Review. Accessed 22 September 2023.

"His Inventions." *Musee Louis Braille*, Musee Louis Braille, no date, museelouisbraille.com/en/ses-inventions. Accessed 18 Feb. 2024.

Janson, Jonathan. "Essential Vermeer 3.0: All Things Vermeer." *Essential Vermeer*, www.essentialvermeer.com. Accessed 19 Feb. 2024.

Jong, Monica, et al. "The Role of Myopia in 2020 Uncorrected Global Visual Impairment." *Investigative Ophthalmology & Visual Science*, The Association for Research in Vision and

Ophthalmology, 1 June 2022, iovs.arvojournals.org/article.aspx?articleid=2779141. Accessed 20 Feb 2024.

Kalantzis, Mary, and Bill Copes. "Lévi-Strauss on the Functions of Writing." *New Learning Online*, no date. newlearningonline.com/literacies/chapter-1/levi-strauss-on-the-functions-of-writing. Accessed 18 Feb. 2024.

Lévi-Strauss, Claude. *Tristes Tropiques*. Penguin Books, 1976.

Maher, Clare. "Myopia Is Responsible for around One-Third of Global Uncorrectable Visual Impairment." *Myopia Profile*, 10 July 2022, www.myopiaprofile.com/articles/myopia-is-re-sponsible-for-around-one-third-of-global-uncorrectable-visual-impairment. Accessed 20 Feb. 2024.

McDermott, Terry. *101 Theory Drive: A Neuroscientist's Quest for Memory*. Vintage, 2010.

Mellor, C. Michael. *Louis Braille: A Touch of Genius*. National Braille Press, 2006.

"National Institute for Blind Youth." *Musee Louis Braille*, Musee Louis Braille, no date. museelouisbraille.com/en/insti-tut-des-jeunes-aveugles. Accessed 18 Feb. 2024.

Perez, David, et al. "Myopic Choroidal Neovascularization." *EyeNet Magazine*, American Academy of Ophthalmology, Mar. 2020, www.aao.org/eyenet/article/myopic-choroi-dal-neovascularization. Accessed 9 Feb 2024.

Rosten, Leo (Author), Ro Blechman (Illustrator), and Lawrence Bush (Editor). *The New Joys of Yiddish*. Harmony, 2010.

Sacks, Oliver. *The Mind's Eye*. Alfred A. Knopf, 2010.

Shah, Vinay A., et al. "Pathologic Myopia (Myopic Degenera-tion)." Edited by Jason Hsu, *EyeWiki*, American Academy of Ophthalmology, 26 Nov. 2023, eyewiki.aao.org/Pathologic_Myopia_(Myopic_Degeneration). Accessed 19 Feb. 2024.

Snyder, Laura J. *Eye of the Beholder: Johannes Vermeer, Antoni van Leeuwenhoek, and the Reinvention of Seeing.* W. W. Norton and Company, 2015.

Social Security Administration. "If You're Blind or Have Low Vision—How We Can Help." *SSA.gov.* Social Security Administration, January 2024. www.ssa.gov/pubs/EN-05-10052. pdf. Accessed 9 Feb. 2024.

Solnit, Rebecca. "Cyclopedia of an Arctic Expedition." in *The Encyclopedia of Trouble and Spaciousness.* Trinity University Press, 2014.

Vellucci, Justin. "Local Rabbi Creates Braille Torah for the Visually Impaired." *Jewish Chronicle of Israel*, Pittsburgh Jewish Chronicle, 1 June 2021, jewishchronicle.timesofisrael.com/ local-rabbi-creates-braille-torah-for-the-visually-impaired. Accessed 17 Feb. 2024.

Vimont, Celia. "Eye Chart Facts and History." *American Academy of Ophthalmology,* March 4, 2022, www.aao.org/eye-health/tips-prevention/eye-chart-facts-history. Accessed 11 Feb. 2024.

"WHO launches First World Report on Vision." *World Health Organization,* 8 Oct. 2019. www.who.int/news/item/08-10-2019-who-launches-first-world-report-on-vision. Accessed 26 Feb. 2024.

Wilson, Kimberley, and Xand van Tulleken. "The Eyes." *Made of Stronger Stuff*, BBC Radio 4, 30 June 2021. bbc.co.uk/pro-grammes/p0957q54. Accessed 18 Feb. 2024.

Wykoff, Charles C. "Pathologic Myopia [Image]." *ONE Network*, American Academy of Ophthalmology, 19 Oct. 2022, www.aao.org/education/image/pathologic-myopia. Accessed 20 Feb 2024.

Yap, Aaron, and Jay J. Meyer. "Degenerative Myopia." *StatPearls [Internet].*, U.S. National Library of Medicine, 19 Sept. 2022, www.ncbi.nlm.nih.gov/books/NBK574560. Accessed 19 Feb. 2024.

Yong, Ed. *An Immense World: How Animal Senses Reveal the Hidden Realms Around Us*. Random House, 2022.

Acknowledgments

Thank you to the publications who have published earlier versions of these pieces, including:

Baltimore Review: "Entries from *The Braille Encyclopedia,*" a lyric essay constructed, in part, of: "Blind," "Blinds," "Blood," "Body," and "Braille"

Dust and Fire: "Marriage," as a prose poem titled "What Remained"

Nimrod International Journal of Prose & Poetry: "Yearning," as a poem titled "You Can't Get Back"

Poetry: "Awl" and "Cell"

Touch the Donkey: "Blue," "Contraction," "Ointment," "Synesthesia," "Touch," and "Umami"

Many thanks to the following arts organizations, fellowships, and residencies:

A 2015 Metropolitan Regional Arts Council Next Step Fund Grant made possible the explorations of essay form that ultimately led to this book.

A 2018 Minnesota State Arts Board Artist Initiative grant supported completion of *The Braille Encyclopedia.*

A 2023 McKnight Artist Fellowship in Writing—administered by the Loft Literary Center and selected by judge Alexander Chee—made possible the revision of *The Braille Encyclopedia* into its final form.

To Jerod Santek and everyone at Write On, Door County; to Amy Weber and all the people and other beings at Bloedel Reserve; to Chantal Harris, Chef Lulu Ranta, and all the staff, townspeople, and fellow artists at Monson Arts; and to the Christine Center.

So many people helped in so many ways to make this book possible. If I were even partly comprehensive, this would be the most encyclopedic part of the book. But please know, I'm thinking of you as I list some categories of gratitude:

Thanks to the team at Rose Metal Press, especially to Abby Beckel and Kathleen Rooney, for their ambitious vision for this book and for their years of leadership and commitment to publishing that expands the possibilities of writing beyond easy categories. I have loved and learned so much from the other authors and titles they've brought into the world and am delighted to join their company.

Thanks to many writer friends who generously provided sage feedback on parts or all of various incarnations of the manuscript or otherwise offered support or resources which helped me imagine, write, re-imagine, and re-rewrite this book. You are too numerous to name, but special thanks to Carolyn Williams-Noren for multiple nuanced reads and to Morgan Grayce Willow, for being such a wonderful guide in my first explorations of essay, which led, in such an essayistic way, to this book.

Thanks also to the many people whose conversations helped me better understand the topics of this book, including Scott Artley, John Lee Clark, Kerstin Gorham, Tara Inmon, Lisa Larges, Joya Musa, Kelly McCrary, and Cindy Smith.

Thanks to these teachers and colleagues for prompts, fostering community, and other resources that led to specific pieces in this work:

Rebecca Brown, 2016 Minnesota Northwoods Writers Conference (MNWC): "Cobbler"

Jess Franken, First Pancake Club: "Academia," "Kindness," "Oyg," and "Yellow"

Caryn Miriam Goldberg: "Yearning," from the springboard of Sharon Olds' "I Go Back to May 1937"

J. Drew Lanham, (2021 MNWC): "Motivation" and "Zorro"

Kalyani Madhu: "Quipu," for sharing her deep history-of-mathematics expertise.

MaryAnn Moenck: "Oyg," for digging up those newspaper clippings about my family.

Thanks also to those who first read the work as strangers—workshop instructors and participants, judges and panelists, and literary magazine editors, whose comments, publications, and awards or encouraging rejection notes all made a difference.

Thanks to the broader circle of my writing communities: the fellow writers and artists who anchor me in my creative life. To Karen Hering and Ranae Hanson, my writing sisters and partners in getting and keeping to the tasks of our writing. To the Ginger Poets, my long-time writing group, who graciously continue to read my work even as I've wandered deeper and deeper into prose-land. To Jess Franken and the incredibly brilliant and generous writers she convened in 2023, thank you First Pancake Club/Coven. Thanks to the staff, faculty, and fellow writers of the Minnesota Northwoods Writers Conference; that annual gathering on the shores of Lake Bemidji is a testament to the possibilities of combining craft, a concern for justice, and creative community.

Thank you to the people who have gifted me with their trust and words in the poetry workshops I lead in so many community settings, both through my Known By Heart project and through COMPAS.

Thanks to the organizations who make so much reading accessible, especially to Bookshare and the National Library Service for the Blind and Print Disabled (with special gratitude to my state network library, Minnesota Braille Talking Books), and State Services for the Blind Communications Center.

Thanks to the programs that have helped me re-learn to read, write, and move through the world, empowering me and many others to live our fullest possible lives. Big thanks to the staff, fellow students, and instructors of Vision Loss Resources. I learned so much from you all. Special thanks again to Cindy Smith and Kelly McCrary, as well as to Jean Christy and Lisa Butler. Thanks also to Minnesota State Services for the Blind, especially my dedicated vocational counselors, Annie Fradella and Stephen Larson.

Thanks to Jen Elmquist, Lucinda Pepper, and Lisa Froehling for guiding me in the body, mind, and life work that provides the ground on which creative work becomes possible.

And thanks to my family, the living and the dead, the biological and the bonus. Gratitude and love to Ray—stand up and be seen if you're willing.

About the Author

Naomi Cohn is a writer and teaching artist whose work explores reclamation. Her past includes a childhood among Chicago academics; involvement in a guerrilla feminist art collective; and work as an encyclopedia copy editor, community organizer, grant writer, fundraising consultant, and therapist. A 2023 McKnight Artist Fellow in Writing, her previous publications include a chapbook, *Between Nectar & Eternity* (Red Dragonfly Press, 2013), and pieces in *Baltimore Review, Fourth River, Hippocampus, Terrain,* and *Poetry,* among others. Cohn has also appeared on NPR and been honored by a Best of the Net Finalist and two Pushcart nominations. Raised in Chicago, she now lives on unceded Dakota territory in Saint Paul, Minnesota.

A Note About the Type

Typography decisions for *The Braille Encyclopedia* were made with optimal readability in mind, to make it as accessible as possible for readers with low vision. The title on the cover is set in Optician Sans, designed by the Norwegian company ANTI Hamar and the typographer Fábio Duarte Martins in November 2018. The design was inspired by historical eye charts, which measure vision clarity. The braille font below the title is a free typeface simply called Braille. The interior display text is set in Atkinson Hyperlegible, a sans serif font that was designed to be maximally legible to low vision readers. It was developed in a collaboration between the Braille Institute of America—after whose founder J. Robert Atkinson it is named—and Applied Design Works, and was made freely available in 2019. Font families are typically designed with a focus on uniformity, which can make distinguishing between similar letterforms difficult for those with vision issues. In contrast, the individual letters in Atkinson Hyperlegible were designed with clear differentiation of forms in mind. Finally, the body text of *The Braille Encyclopedia* is set in Georgia, a clear and readable serif font. It was designed by Matthew Carter and released by Microsoft in 1996. Many major newspapers use Georgia for their body text because of its high legibility, including *The New York Times* and *The Guardian*. It has a taller x-height—the distance between the baseline and the mean line of lowercase letters—than other classic serifs, and a slightly thicker stroke, which makes it easier to read at small sizes.

—Heather Butterfield